HOW TO
SUCCEED
AS A
HEALTHCARE
LEADER

HOW TO
SUCCEED
AS A
HEALTHCARE
LEADER

RACHEL MILLER, MD

publish
your gift

HOW TO SUCCEED AS A HEALTHCARE LEADER
Copyright © 2022 Rachel Miller
All rights reserved.

Published by Publish Your Gift®
An imprint of Purposely Created Publishing Group, LLC

Names mentioned in this book have been changed to protect confidentiality.

Printed in the United States of America

ISBN: 978-1-64484-581-3 (print)
ISBN: 978-1-64484-582-0 (ebook)

Special discounts are available on bulk quantity purchases by book clubs, associations and special interest groups. For details email: sales@publishyourgift.com or call (888) 949-6228.
For information log on to www.PublishYourGift.com

DEDICATION

This book is dedicated to my husband, Casey, and
to my two daughters, Victoria and Autumn.

TABLE OF CONTENTS

INTRODUCTION

Throughout the years, I have had interactions with many healthcare systems, both as an employee and as a patient.

When I was just thirteen, I underwent surgery, where I developed a relationship with the physician who cared for me. He was so kind, answering all my questions and helping me not to be afraid. I wanted to be a doctor just like him.

I immediately started my journey to become a physician. I switched high schools to attend a science magnet school and studied hard to get the grades I would need to get into a great college. Despite having teachers who doubted if I would be able to make it, I was successful.

I went to an incredible university, North Carolina State. While there, I applied myself and was able to do well and get into medical school.

In medical school, there were countless sleepless and stressful nights. I was afraid of failure and worried that I would not make it. Despite all this, I persevered and was able to graduate from medical school and make it to residency.

After successfully completing residency and landing a dream job as an obstetrician and gynecologist, I had the satisfaction of knowing that all my hard work had paid off.

I essentially spent my whole life trying to get to the point where I could take care of others independently. Today, I have many friends who are nurses and fellow physicians. A majority of these friends love the science and art of medicine. They love caring for their patients. But they are growing more and more frustrated with medicine because of the direction in which healthcare is going. I agree.

America is currently in a healthcare crisis. These are unprecedented times. The problems in the healthcare system are not problems that a consultant can solve. It is not a situation where any one person knows the answer to every organization's problem. The solution will take the leadership efforts of everyone in the field of healthcare.

Leadership happens in boardrooms and administrative offices. It happens on clinical teams. It happens in the example of every healthcare worker who leads through the application of their own excellence.

All of us who are passionate about patient care and have the skills to do the job will need to be involved as we look for ways to improve and implement those changes.

As this happens, some of us will step up to management and executive leadership roles. It is going to take coaching to help these new leaders realize the perfect answers to their problems.

I am one of the physicians who has moved into a leadership position. I want to help America get out of its current crisis, and I see this as an opportunity to bring what I know as a physician to bear in a new way.

So, I worked hard to learn new skills and get to the point where I am now—helping healthcare leaders and executives to lead in a more authentic way. I believe that authentic leadership—leadership based on ethical behavior, transparent sharing of information, and meaningful two-way communication—is vital to the future of healthcare. It is the only way healthcare providers can continue to love practicing medicine.

Today, I am a board-certified obstetrician and gynecologist. I am also a certified executive coach and a Dr. John Maxwell leadership coach, speaker, and trainer. For the past decade, I have devoted my career to eliminating the disconnect between physicians and organizational leaders in the healthcare industry.

I have experienced this disconnect firsthand. Soon after I started practicing medicine in 2009, I had the opportunity to become involved in the management and business sides of the practice. But to many of my colleagues, taking this step meant I had "joined the dark side." They saw the business side of medicine as "us versus them."

I understand why this is. As a physician, I have had to deal with challenges like the pressure to see more patients per day and the burden of dealing with new, imperfect electronic health record (EHR) systems. My situation is not unique. Many of my colleagues deal with the same challenges.

It often seemed that the business of medicine was making it hard to practice medicine. But in my leadership role, I have also seen that we all wanted to provide good healthcare.

Business and management training is not a standard part of medical education. Medical training is not part of business school. A lack of mutual understanding is endemic. And this disconnect between physicians and healthcare leaders is an obstacle in dealing with the very real problems of the healthcare system.

The COVID-19 pandemic has stressed the healthcare system dramatically. As the disease swept across the country, emergency rooms were taxed beyond capacity, elective procedures were postponed, and doctors and nurses reported burnout in record numbers. Then, while public debate raged about the need for vaccination, hospitalization and deaths rose again as the Delta variant swept through areas where people remained unvaccinated.

At the best of times, patient care can be physically and emotionally demanding. Physicians have the highest suicide rate among all professions, and the suicide rate for nurses is higher than that for the general public.

During COVID-19, stress levels soared due to the need to remain gowned, gloved, and masked at all times while working extraordinarily long hours with critically ill patients to deal with an epidemic disease (Flores 2021).

COVID-19 is stressing the system and challenging medical professionals in ways we have not seen before. But the challenge of COVID-19 is made much worse because it has exposed problems that have been percolating for decades. These are fundamental issues that result in a healthcare system that is inefficient, expensive, frustrating for patients, and disheartening for dedicated physicians and other caregivers.

Statistics that compare the United States to other high-income countries show that our healthcare system has significant problems. The United States spends twice as much per person on healthcare yet has the lowest life expectancy and the highest rate of suicide. We have fewer doctors per person, resulting in fewer doctor visits per person each year. And our obesity and chronic disease rates are twice as high (Tikkanen and Abrams 2020).

Some of the specific challenges we need to address to solve these problems include:

- Unequal access to healthcare—This is a complex problem that involves economic, racial, and ethnic disparities. Among many indicators of the problem:
  - * Infant mortality for black babies is 2.3–2.5 times greater than for white babies.
  - * The rate of diabetes for Native Americans and Latinos is 30 percent higher than for whites.
  - * Blacks and Latinos are more likely to be uninsured, resulting in less access to healthcare and less preventive care.

* Minorities experience bias in how care is provided due to the fact that minorities represent a much smaller percentage of the health profession workforce than of the general population (Ely 2020; Riley 2012).

- Flawed implementation of EHRs—Despite the promise of EHRs to improve patient care and make medicine more efficient and cost-effective, we have systems that are expensive, difficult to use, and unable to communicate with each other:

  * EHR implementation costs hundreds of thousands of dollars for medical practices and millions of dollars for hospitals.

  * Physicians who move from one practice to another typically need to learn at least one completely different EHR system. These systems are not intuitive and require a huge learning curve.

  * Often, different departments in the same hospital use EHRs that cannot share data with each other (Patel 2019).

- An epidemic of chronic disease—According to the Centers for Disease Control and Prevention (CDC), 90 percent of our healthcare dollars are used to treat the effects of diabetes, hypertension, and other chronic diseases. Yet many of these problems are preventable or can be significantly reduced by better healthcare (CDC 2019).

- Administrative and regulatory burdens—Hospitals and medical practices must deal with separate reporting systems for public insurance and for each type of private insurance. Hospitals and other healthcare providers must report compliance with 629 separate regulations from just four of the federal agencies with regulatory authority over healthcare (Kaplan and Abongwa 2020).

It will take the involvement of everyone in healthcare to solve these problems. This means that leadership at all levels of healthcare is a critical component in addressing the situation. Physicians must be part of the mix.

That is what this book is about: the importance of physician leadership and the essential skills of good leaders. We will talk about excellence, the problem of burnout, developing leadership skills, understanding yourself as a person and a leader, the role of emotional intelligence, the strength that comes from gratitude, the value of community and mentors, the importance of connections, and the coaching approach to leadership.

As a medical professional myself, I understand the complexities of our healthcare system. I know the depth of compassion and commitment my colleagues bring to their work. And I appreciate the level of excellence we each strive to achieve. That is where I would like to start.

CHAPTER I

A PASSION FOR EXCELLENCE

Successful leaders are passionate about what they do.

Why? What is passion?

Inward, passion is energy and intense interest. It is a motivator for achievement.

Outward, passion is magnetic. It is an expression of dedication and enthusiasm that inspires others to join you.

I think it is interesting that the word *passion* comes from the Latin root *pati*, to suffer. (Mohana 2016). At first this seems wrong, but it makes sense when you think about it because passion is a source of energy and drive that can propel you through things that are tough.

The more passionate you are about something, the more you care. The more you care, the more motivated you will be, the more effort you will put in, and the greater the satisfaction when you succeed. We all know this from experience.

It was my passion that got me through my medical training.

When I was in medical school, my most heartbreaking experience was finding out that I did not pass a major national exam. I had spent countless hours studying for this exam. I missed family events and get-togethers with friends. I missed birthday parties—all so I could study hard to prepare for the exam.

Even so, I missed the passing score by just a couple of points. Initially, I was devastated and quite honestly wondered if I was doing the right thing in life.

After this failure, I confess I spent a little time wallowing in my sadness. But I soon remembered why I was in medical school. I buckled down and sought help.

I learned that there was a better way to study for this type of test, so I practiced. On the second attempt, I did amazingly well. I improved my score tremendously and was able to continue on my journey to become a physician.

Despite failing that exam, I remembered that I was in medical school because I wanted to learn how to become a doctor so I could take care of people. Without passion, I would not have been able to overcome such a major setback.

That failure taught me so many things. I learned how to study for such an exam. I learned that I could succeed even if I failed the first time. And I was reminded of what perseverance could help me accomplish.

Without passion, there is no perseverance. From then on, I was able to pass my subsequent exams and realize my dreams.

Now, research is showing how passion works. In one experiment, a group of people was asked to perform tasks. Some of the tasks were interesting (motivating) and others were mundane. During the motivating tasks, everyone showed brain activity in areas associated with feelings of satisfaction and reward-processing (Lee and Reeve 2017). Passion feels good.

Passion is enthusiasm. It is caring. It is excitement and zeal. It is the feeling you have when you get up in the morning and know that there is something meaningful waiting in your day.

Passion is not enough. Knowledge and skill are important, too. But passion is essential.

WHERE DOES PASSION COME FROM?

Like many people who choose healthcare as a career, I had an experience that inspired me with a passion for healing. For some of us, this is the experience of seeing a loved one go through a health crisis. For others like me, the experience is more personal.

My passion for healthcare started when I was a child and needed surgery. I was young. I was scared. And I was greatly helped by the doctor who cared for me.

The doctor was skilled, and the surgery was successful. Just as important, he was so empathetic and kind; he gave me information, he allayed my fears, he helped me be brave, and he inspired me to want to help other people in the same way.

When I was a teenager, I started volunteering at my local hospital. I was able to see what possibilities lay ahead. I continued to volunteer in my local hospital through college, and these experiences fueled my passion for caring for patients.

Initially, I did not want to become a surgeon, but I wanted to care for people as a physician. It was later in my journey that I decided to enter a specialty that does involve some surgery, obstetrics and gynecology (OB/GYN).

That desire, that passion for healing with kindness and empathy, saw me through years of study, internship, residency, and into practice as an OB/GYN. My enthusiasm for my mission to help others fueled long hours of study and rotations through the hospital as an intern and resident.

As an OB/GYN, my passion was rewarded as I applied the lesson I had learned from the physician who treated me as a child. I was able to use my skills with empathy to give both healthy and sick patients the best possible treatment and care.

And that is another aspect of passion, the drive to achieve excellence.

Medicine is challenging. You are dealing with people's lives, and that requires the best you can give.

It was in the spirit of supporting excellence that I took my first steps into leadership.

I mentioned earlier that I had the opportunity to become a part of the management leadership team in my healthcare system. I took that step because I was curious. I understood what it meant to practice good medicine, but I did not really understand the business side. And I knew that this was an area of stress for my colleagues and me.

I wanted to learn about leadership because I was experiencing stress based on management issues I did not fully understand—and also because I was seeing so many tired and burned-out physicians working day in and day out.

I knew that we all wanted to be able to practice the best possible medicine, and I felt that there had to be a way that I could help.

WHAT DOES PASSION LOOK LIKE?

Passion in healthcare wears many different faces.

For one surgeon, passion may focus on the mastery of technique. For another surgeon, it may focus on the ability to repair broken bodies. An internist might be passionate about diagnosis. A nurse might be passionate about communicating clearly with patients who are in pain or confused. An orderly might be passionate about treating patients with dignity when they need help with the activities of daily living.

Passion in the workplace does not have to be boisterous or flashy. Rather, it can be expressed with focus, dedication, confidence, and high-quality work. Passion is the impetus that helps a person handle the unappealing aspects of a job.

Every job has a lot of facets. Some we like better than others. The part we are passionate about is what keeps us going. It is the part that helps us keep a good attitude.

People who are passionate tend to have less stress, and so they have a better attitude.

When I was growing up, my parents taught me the Golden Rule: treat everyone else the way you want to be treated yourself. This is so true. When we treat others well, they often reciprocate. It is the same with attitude. If you present a good attitude, it helps lift the people around you. That is part of leadership.

In healthcare, as in any complex endeavor, it takes the excellence of everyone on a team to achieve the best. This is one of the things I find most rewarding about leadership coaching. We can all be leaders in doing our best.

MAINTAINING YOUR PASSION

No one is "up" all the time. We all have good days and bad days.

To handle my moods and the normal ups and downs of life, I have found that at times, "fake it 'til you make it" is true. No matter how I feel, if I put a smile on my face, it actually helps me feel better.

Putting on a smile will prevent you from spreading your low feelings to others and help you maintain your passion for what you do. It can be an effective way to help you work through internal lows.

In a stressful profession like healthcare, however, there are also external challenges with maintaining your passion. Once you are on the job, even though you are in a position to accomplish your goals, you will encounter emotional, physical, and administrative stresses every day.

I listed some of these stresses in the introduction when talking about the systemic problems affecting our healthcare system. Other stresses are related to the specific aspects of a physician's job, things like:

- chronically or critically ill patients;

- patients with undiagnosed illnesses who rely on you for a cure; and

- clinical problems you cannot just forget about at the end of the workday.

In addition to preventive medicine and wellness care, doctors deal with critical issues of life and death. They are constantly making decisions. It is a matter of balancing what you know with what is possible with what the patient wants—all while dealing with issues that could have a long-lasting impact on a patient's life.

One important thing you can do to maintain your passion in the face of these challenges is to be aware of every win. What may seem like a small win to you can make a big difference in a patient's life. Success provides momentum to keep you going.

Surround yourself with like-minded people. As an employee, you do not choose your coworkers. What you can do, however, is create a circle of positivity around yourself.

Being a leader does not necessarily mean being a boss. You can also be a leader through the example that you set. I have seen offices where it was a member of the medical staff, not the administrative boss, who was the de facto leader of the team.

As a leader, you have the power to affect how your colleagues feel and help them do the best they can. This will fuel your passion, too. (I will talk more about this in Chapter 7.)

And finally, stay curious and engaged. My passion for providing the kind of healthcare I received as a child inspired me to become a physician. Then once I started practicing, my curiosity about how the healthcare system worked, combined with my passion for supporting excellence in patient care, led me into management.

The more I learned about management and leadership, the more I became convinced that this was the best way for me to follow my passion. I realized that we cannot solve the problems we face in our healthcare system unless we are able to bridge the gap between physicians and nonphysician leadership. And so, I became a healthcare executive and leadership coach.

Now, through my company, Pocket Bridges, LLC, I am able to spend every day helping physicians like myself, as well as nonclinical administrators and managers, become effective leaders of their teams in providing excellent healthcare.

CHAPTER 2

COMBATING BURNOUT

The burnout caused by COVID-19 has pushed an already stressed industry to the breaking point. Many physicians have experienced or are currently experiencing burnout. This is something we are hearing much more about now than in years past. It has caused physicians and also nurses to leave medicine in droves (Hu and Dill 2021).

I am a part of many different physician and nonphysician groups where burnout is a constant topic. Fortunately, more and more conversations are being had around burnout, which is encouraging because it brings this problem to the fore.

Burnout is one way that healthcare is changing and will forever be changed by the impact of the COVID-19 pandemic disease.

But physicians were already stressed by deep-seated problems in our healthcare system.

Daily, they face situations that they feel are impossible to change. For instance, we are being asked to do things that are against what we feel is our moral obligation as medical caregivers. This causes distress. I call it moral injury. Along with so many of my physician colleagues, I have experienced it myself.

On the one hand, we physicians feel that we have a moral obligation to do our best, to take the best care of our patients, and to avoid causing harm to our patients (as we pledged in the oath we took when entering medical school).

On the other hand, there are pressures to keep patient satisfaction high while at the same time seeing more and more patients per day, every day, and to limit the cost of the care that is being provided.

These pressures inherently cause a conflict that we live with on a daily basis.

There was already a shortage of doctors in the US healthcare system caused by the combination of retirements among an aging physician population and a congressional cap on the number of residency positions that are available every year to train new physicians (AAMC 2021; Wofford 2020).

Now with COVID-19, younger physicians are also quitting medicine in record numbers.

As reported in the *New York Times*, safety is now an issue because personal protective equipment can be hard to secure, especially for private practices. Patients are angry and afraid, and these emotions often bubble over on healthcare providers. Thousands of medical practices have closed or plan to close. Older doctors in large medical systems are retiring early or looking for less stressful jobs. Other, younger doctors have had to take a break and do not know if they will go back (Abelson 2020).

There is also a crisis in the nursing profession. Even before COVID-19, starting in 2012, the healthcare system in the US was experiencing a nursing shortage. More and more registered nurses were seeking higher education in order to move out of direct patient care and into more lucrative roles such as nurse anesthetist and nurse practitioner. Although that workforce is needed, there have not been enough new nurses entering the profession to take on the front-facing roles that are also needed. And in addition, the aging baby boomer generation is increasing the need for nurses to work in home healthcare, as well as primary and urgent care (Behring 2021).

These are complex problems, and they cannot be solved without the involvement of physicians and nurses. The people on the front lines of providing care need to have a voice in deciding the best way to provide that care.

Through coaching and leadership development, we can start to move the needle in a different direction.

It will take effective leaders to address the problems in our healthcare system. Effective leaders understand the range of activities needed in that system. Coaching helps create effective leaders by providing actionable feedback to them on the job while leadership skills are being honed.

THE IMPORTANCE OF PHYSICIAN LEADERSHIP

When I accepted the directorship of my clinical department, several of my colleagues joked that I was going to the dark side. It was so frustrating. I was a doctor just like them, but all of a sudden, it felt like I was the enemy.

Clinical leaders are a fundamental part of any healthcare organization. Clinical leaders in management who understand medicine are essential.

There are many sources of evidence that support having physicians as part of the management leadership team. This is because the physician's expert knowledge of the organization's primary goal improves the overall performance of the healthcare organization:

- A *Harvard Business Review* study reported that the best hospitals, as ranked by the *US News & World Report*, all have physicians in the C-suite (Stoller et al. 2016).

- The same Harvard study cited research that finds that the most significant factor in hospital management practices and performance is a higher proportion of managers who have a clinical degree.

Why does having physicians in leadership positions matter? To again cite the Harvard study, a physician leader lends credibility. A physician understands the essential requirements of the institution's core mission. This inspires trust in the medical team. It also makes it easier to design and implement systems that measure meaningful aspects of patient care and to use those indicators to improve performance.

It is unfortunate that two of the ways success is measured in medicine today—performance and value—can mitigate against high-quality patient care if they are not applied appropriately.

Performance matters, but performance needs to be measured in terms of patient outcomes, not in terms of the number of patients treated. And when outcomes depend both on how sick the patient is as well as the quality of care received, performance can be challenging to measure.

Value matters, too, but value in the medical industry is not the same as reducing costs.

In an environment where healthcare providers are pressured to see more and more patients, it is understandable that "value" can seem like a dirty word. I think this is why so many of my colleagues reacted negatively when I moved into leadership. They knew and trusted me, but they did not trust the system.

It is unfortunate that performance and value measures were introduced into medicine by businesspeople, not clinicians. Why does this matter? Let me share a story I heard from a friend in another industry that illustrates what I mean.

A woman named Shayna ran the video division of a company that had previously served only internal clients. Now the company wanted to expand into external production work. Video production is not nearly as complex as medicine, but the dynamics of measurement systems are the same.

In order to get external clients, the company hired a salesman and reorganized the other eleven staff members. At the direction of company management, the salesman worked on commission, and the two lead producers got bonuses based on the number of videos they produced. Everyone else's salary remained the same. Commission and bonuses were tracked through the company's financial software.

The first year was slow, as often happens when starting a new business. At the end of the year, the salesman was unhappy because he did not make as much money as he wanted due to lower-than-hoped sales. The lead producers liked getting a bonus, but the rest of the staff were unhappy because they had been part of the teams that produced each video.

So, at the start of the second year, Shayna—the producer and leader of the production group—asked the management to change the incentive structure. Management agreed.

The salesman got a salary against commission. The lead producers still got bonuses based on their client base. But Shayna wanted the incentive structure to recognize everyone's contributions to the team's overall success, and so bonuses were also extended to all other staff members: the receptionist, the office manager, and everyone else on the production team. These bonus amounts were based on the production group's ability to exceed their profitability targets.

The result? The entire team learned what it took to be a profitable business as well as do good work, and both growth and profitability skyrocketed.

It was Shayna who understood this business and was able to recommend an incentive structure that worked.

This example is very relevant to the situation we face today in healthcare. When physicians and other healthcare workers become involved as leaders, healthcare systems can evolve to be sound businesses *and* provide excellent patient care.

THE CHALLENGE OF PHYSICIAN LEADERSHIP

Excellent clinical skills give physicians credibility among their peers, but medical training does not give physicians leadership skills.

To become effective leaders in complex, dynamic healthcare organizations, physicians also need social skills and a solid understanding of the value of their administration and management. These things are not a routine part of the medical school or residency curriculum.

In an article in the *Harvard Business Review*, Dr. Thomas Lee summarized the disconnect between physician training and the managerial needs of today's healthcare systems (Lee 2010). As Dr. Lee explains it, older physicians who have been tapped to move into management and leadership roles were trained at a time when the doctor was in charge. Doctors were expected to work long hours and be hands-on through all phases of their patients' care.

But medicine today is focused on patient-centered care. And as healthcare has become more and more high-tech, a system has developed in which there are many medical specialties that each have a voice in patient care and have separate administrative structures.

Navigating leadership and effecting change in this environment requires a collaborative approach. It takes teamwork to improve performance.

In the nexus between clinical patient care goals, hospital and practice business goals, insurance requirements, and the government's regulatory priorities, it will take a concerted effort by strong, physician-led teams with a passion for realizing the promise of providing the best possible patient care.

This will greatly reduce stress and help relieve the problem of burnout.

WAYS TO DEAL WITH STRESS

There are several things you can do right now that will ameliorate the effects of stress. These include treatments such as chiropractic adjustment and acupuncture, and energy healing such as Reiki, yoga, tai chi, and meditation. It is a measure of the value of these therapies that the National Center for Complementary and Integrative Health

(NCCIH) of the National Institutes of Health has found evidence of their effectiveness (NCCIH 2020). Meta-analyses have shown that when used as monotherapy as well as adjunctive therapy, both yoga and mindfulness-based meditation can improve depression and anxiety. The most helpful intervention found in this meta-analysis was exercise (Saeed 2019).

Coaching can help, too. I offer executive leadership coaching, but there are also various other types of coaching. Some coaches focus specifically on burnout, and several studies substantiate the value of this type of coaching.

Today, both physicians and nurses experiencing burnout are seeking help through coaching. A recent article in the *Journal of the American Medical Association* (JAMA) showed participants' increased resilience and quality of life and decreased emotional exhaustion and overall burnout in relation to coaching. This study demonstrated that with coaching, there was a decrease in the participants' emotional exhaustion by 19.5 percent. Additionally, burnout decreased by 17 percent. Resilience increased by 20.3 percent, and quality of life improved by 4.2 percent. These results were demonstrated with just six months of coaching (Dyrbye et al. 2019).

Several other studies have been published that have similar results. For example, in the *Journal of Occupational Health Psychology*, a study showed that after just six coaching sessions with primary care physicians, there was increased engagement, improved psychological capital, improved job satisfaction, and decreased burnout (McGonagle et al. 2020).

THE IMPORTANCE OF ADDRESSING CONTRIBUTORS OF BURNOUT

At the end of 2020, the medical information website Medscape reported that overall burnout among physicians was 42 percent. This was relatively unchanged from 2019, but in addition, 20 percent fewer physicians reported being happy with their work and life overall. They said that burnout was having a negative impact on their personal lives, mental health, and ability to provide good patient care. And significantly, only 8 percent of the physicians pointed to COVID-19 as the primary cause of their burnout (Medscape 2021).

Burnout is exacerbated by COVID-19, but it has been a problem for decades.

The World Health Organization (WHO) is changing the definition of burnout from a "state of vital exhaustion" to a "syndrome conceptualized as resulting from chronic workplace stress that has not been successfully managed." It clearly defines burnout as an occupational hazard rather than a medical issue.

There are five main causes of burnout (Clark 2019):

1. the frustrations of EHR implementation
2. the constant introduction of new medical technologies

3. long hours
4. financial stress
5. bureaucracy and loss of control

Change cannot happen if we do not deal with the issues that are causing burnout for so many physicians, nurses, and other healthcare staff. Let's consider some of these and the kinds of actions that will be necessary to resolve them.

Poorly Designed EHR Workflow

When electronic health records (EHRs) were introduced, the government did nothing to help ensure that EHR technology would work seamlessly across the many different healthcare organizations. We saw the importance of this kind of government action during the introduction of color television.

All color televisions, no matter the manufacturer, were required to be compatible with existing black and white television technology. But in the name of the free market, the government did not require a national standard for EHRs.

The result has been an operational nightmare.

Doctors spend nearly six hours a day entering data or otherwise interacting with EHRs. This is nearly twice as much time as they spend on direct patient care (Arndt et al. 2017). This is totally antithetical to quality patient care.

Efforts are being made to address the problem. Many healthcare systems now provide medical scribes to do the work of data entry, significantly increasing costs. Research studies are testing proposals for ways to make EHR systems easier and less time-consuming to use (Sinsky et al. 2020).

EHR technology has great promise to improve the efficiency of healthcare by making complete patient medical records available to every healthcare provider. But these systems need to support, not hamper, clinical operations.

Physicians have an important role to play in defining how EHRs can fit most effectively into the workflow of patient care.

Constant Introduction of New Medical Technologies

In recent decades, the story of medical science has been a story of new technologies to improve diagnosis and care: pacemakers, MRIs, dialysis, PillCams, joint replacements, stents, robotic surgery—there are more and more tools being made available to medical science.

But every new technology comes with a learning curve, and the information available from new diagnostic tools must be evaluated and understood.

Physicians have a role to play in deciding how new technologies can best be applied to improve patient care.

Long Hours

Doctors have always worked long hours. This can be unavoidable, but there is a significant difference between time spent on patient care and time spent on other tasks like EHRs or regulatory compliance reporting.

Physicians and other healthcare staff need just as much sleep as everyone else, but the reality of medicine is that illnesses do not follow a nine-to-five schedule.

Only someone who understands medical science can decide when it is appropriate for a clinician to stay on-site during the course of treatment and when a patient's care can safely be transferred to the hands of another shift.

One result of working long hours is sleep deprivation. Another can be poor work-life balance. Both cause stress.

Financial Stress

A major source of financial stress is student debt. Student debt is not elusive to physicians. But it is expensive to become a doctor, and most medical students graduate with an enormous average debt of more than $190,000 (Clark 2019).

In addition, because we are a litigious society, doctors must also deal with liability issues. The high cost of malpractice insurance causes financial stress—not to mention the emotional stress of a potential lawsuit.

Bureaucracy and Loss of Control

One of the major changes in the practice of medicine has been in the role of the physician.

Doctors used to be the heroes, the main decision-makers when it came to patient care. Now, decisions about patient care are influenced by a host of technical specialists, insurance companies, government regulation, and the resulting bureaucracy.

Health insurance increases patient access to care. Insured people are more likely to have regular checkups, wellness, and preventive care. But insurance company rules can also have an enormous negative impact on the practice of medicine.

One example of how insurance affects care is the step therapy rule for cancer treatment. The rule requires doctors to start chemotherapy treatments with drugs chosen by the insurance company rather than the physician. Insurance companies almost always choose the least expensive option, even when that drug is more toxic than the doctor thinks is needed, or even when it was already tried—without success—at a time when the patient was covered by a different insurance plan. These bureaucratic, not medical, decisions can be very costly—even deadly— for a patient (Patt 2020).

Other insurance company rules that affect care include:

- requiring prior authorization (i.e., an approval form that the physician must file with the insurer) before a patient can get a particular medication or treatment;

- excluding medications based on the cost or a lack of financial incentive from the pharmaceutical company to the insurer;

- switching the medication prescribed by the doctor to a similar—but not necessarily as effective—medication chosen by the insurance company; and

- extremely low reimbursement for mental health services (Ginsberg 2017).

These limitations are especially stressful when physicians know that decisions are being made based on factors not directly related to a patient's condition.

Malpractice insurance also affects the practice of medicine in ways that extend beyond medical malfeasance.

Insurance costs can be very high for the riskiest specialties, such as surgery, emergency room medicine, and obstetrics. These are specialties where the line is closest between the science of medicine and the art of medicine.

In the early 2000s, there was a crisis of rising malpractice insurance costs, especially for my specialty, OB/GYN. Obstetrics is one of the most expensive specialties to insure. Pregnancy is risky, and new parents can be quick to look for blame if something goes wrong.

Between 2000 and 2003, insurance costs for OB/GYNs went through the roof. In New Jersey, for example, the average cost of premiums went from $34,617 to $78,818. Some doctors stopped caring for high-risk pregnancies or even stopped delivering babies (Donlen and Puro 2003).

In response, some states stepped in with tort reform to limit the insurance costs and liability, and the cost of malpractice insurance stabilized. In subsequent years, insurance premium costs have even gone down (Belk 2020).

Malpractice lawsuits, however, are extremely stressful, even if the physician is judged to have done their job correctly.

Medicine is both a science and an art. Despite the ever-growing technical options for diagnosis and treatment, there are limits to what medicine can do. These limits alone are a source of stress for physicians because not every patient can be cured.

CHAPTER 3

DEVELOPING PROFESSIONAL AND LEADERSHIP SKILLS

I saw a story on the website of Relias Media, the continuing medical education company, that illustrates different ways that leadership matters in improving healthcare (Relias Media 2000).

Aileen Day, the director of medical management at North Shore Medical Center Union Hospital in Lynn, Massachusetts, wanted to counsel a pulmonologist, Dr. Jain, whose patients had the longest average length of stay.

From a medical point of view, you want a patient to be able to stay in the hospital as long as necessary for good care, but it is also true that the sooner a patient can go home, the better.

Ms. Day first approached the problem by going to Dr. Jain with the data about the length of stay for all pulmonologists. Rather than telling him, "You need to do better," she challenged the doctor by appealing to his competitive instincts and relying on him to figure out how to solve the problem.

Dr. Jain was surprised at first, but seeing the data inspired him to want to do better. Working with the director, he evaluated what was going on. She gave him literature about different care options. He evaluated what he was doing and found several ways that he and his partners could improve, including changing how they handled rounds and finding ways to get test results more promptly.

The average length of stay for Dr. Jain's patients dropped from 10.4 days to 5.2 days, without any decrease in the quality of care or an increase in readmissions.

These results were achieved through good leadership on the part of the director of medical management and the physician.

Leadership is a team sport.

Ms. Day and Dr. Jain collaborated to their mutual benefit. Ms. Day knew that Dr. Jain understood his practice and the needs of his patients better than she did; she wanted him to be invested in finding a solution. Dr. Jain knew that shorter hospital stays are better for patients; so, when Ms. Day showed him the facts, he was motivated to improve.

In addition, Ms. Day's collaborative approach was a good one in light of the fact that a loss of control is a significant contributor to physician burnout.

This is the kind of leadership we need in healthcare.

WHAT ARE THE QUALITIES OF A GOOD LEADER?

We have all heard the expression "a born leader," and yes, some people are very charismatic, and others follow them.

It takes confidence and decisiveness to be a good leader, and physicians tend to have these traits.

Organizational leadership, however, requires more. It requires developing the skills needed to encourage others to do good work, maintain workflow and productivity, and help organizations navigate the business's ups and downs.

Do a Google search, and you will find many lists of the qualities that make for a good leader. An article in *Forbes* magazine lists eleven qualities of successful leaders (Patel 2017). An article in *Inc.* magazine reports ten key leadership skills that were identified in a survey of 300,000 business leaders (Economy 2018).

Interestingly, these and many similar lists are remarkably consistent. Experts generally agree that good leaders have a combination of these qualities:

- Good leaders have honesty and integrity.
- They have a deep understanding of their industries, often being experts themselves either professionally or technically.
- They are effective communicators.
- They articulate a clear and inspiring vision for the future.
- They have perseverance and drive.
- They are good problem solvers—adaptable, flexible, and innovative.

- They cultivate strong networks both inside and outside their organization.

- And they are collaborators, promoting strong teamwork through respect, delegation, workforce development, and encouraging creativity.

These leadership qualities apply across industries.

WHAT DOES GOOD LEADERSHIP LOOK LIKE IN HEALTHCARE TODAY?

The healthcare industry is a high-stakes environment that is rapidly evolving and incredibly stressful. Good leadership must take this into account.

Looking at the challenges facing the healthcare industry today, we can see that skilled and knowledgeable leaders are needed at all levels of the various healthcare organizations, from hospitals to clinics and private practices. This includes upper management, the directors of clinical teams, office management, and individual workers who lead by the influence of their own example.

It will take strong leadership to overcome the challenges of workforce burnout, organizational inefficiency, administrative and regulatory burdens, and inequalities that plague the system. I firmly believe that good leadership in healthcare requires the clinical understanding that physicians bring to the table.

These physician leaders will need a combination of clinical, business, and interpersonal skills.

In cultivating these leaders, the healthcare industry must deal with the legacy of the "command and control" style of leadership that so many doctors learn during their medical training.

It is true that there are clinical situations when it is important for a strong leader to be in control. But it is equally true that in medicine today, there are many more factors involved in medical decision-making than the physician's individual diagnosis.

The factors involved in medical decision-making include the use of high-tech diagnostic tools that require expert interpretation, the need to adhere to reimbursement rules for patients' insurance coverages, the need to follow clinical management procedures, and the requirements of patient involvement (Hajjaj et al. 2010).

Physician leaders will be well-positioned to deal with all of these factors while working toward the goal of providing good, evidence-based medical care.

One advantage that physician leaders have is that they are intimately familiar with both what it takes to practice good medicine and the obstacles to achieving that goal.

Well-regarded physicians will have credibility with their peers. They will also have a thorough understanding of the essential mission of healthcare—treating patients—and so will be able to balance this imperative with other, business-oriented concerns.

Just one example of a problem that physician leaders can help address is EHRs. Effective leaders in healthcare must understand both the potential benefits and the operational weaknesses of EHR systems so that they can help guide their organizations to improve.

Two solutions that are being implemented now are the use of medical scribes to handle the bulk of EHR data entry and the development of task-specific computer apps that facilitate communication between EHRs and provide actionable medical data to clinicians. These are stopgap measures at best, adding layers of work hours to the use of computer systems that were intended to improve data quality and streamline operations.

For the future, leaders will need to be able to apply the lessons learned from the initial implementation of EHR systems in order to adequately evaluate new EHR technologies.

An article on Johns Hopkins University's website describes the challenge of incorporating physicians into organizational leadership beyond their clinical roles (Ercolano 2017). It points to the fact that although medical schools are starting to add business management and leadership courses, these courses are not part of the core curriculum. Some universities offer combined MD/MBA degrees, but enrollment in these programs remains small.

The result is that because physicians are needed in healthcare leadership, excellent clinicians are promoted into these roles without adequate training.

In 2018, the *Journal of Healthcare Leadership* published a research-based model of what healthcare leadership should look like. It is called the Duke Healthcare Leadership Model (Hargett 2017). The model was developed based on literature review, focus groups, and consensus meetings among healthcare professionals. It defines six essential elements of leadership in healthcare:

1. patient-centeredness
2. integrity
3. selfless service
4. teamwork
5. emotional intelligence
6. critical thinking

The model is diagrammed as a circle. Patient-centeredness is at the core. Everything else revolves around that.

As a physician, I agree with this model, and I understand that physician leadership is critical in order to realize it.

I am encouraged by anecdotal evidence that suggests that an increasing number of younger physicians aspire to healthcare leadership. There are many reasons. These include the anticipation of burnout from physicians in the most high-stress specialties, the desire to earn more money, and also the same commitment to high-quality patient care that drew them to medicine in the first place.

WHAT CAN YOU DO TO BECOME A BETTER LEADER?

As a physician leader, you will find that leadership training is mostly outside of books. It takes consistent, daily effort and involves learning from experience.

The first step toward becoming a better leader is recognizing what you will need to learn—and realizing that this is a skill you can improve and that there are ways to do this, even while you are on the job.

If you have a passion for getting involved as a healthcare leader, you will find the energy and enthusiasm to see you through.

Executive coaching is a great way to approach this learning curve. That is what I received when I took on my first leadership role, and it helped me immensely.

I realized that there were things I needed to learn in order to be an effective leader in my practice. But I was not in a position to drop everything and go back to school. After a few internet searches and speaking with a couple of other healthcare colleagues, I decided to invest in a coach. Once I made the decision to hire a coach, I quickly became overwhelmed with questions such as, "How do I pick a coach?" and "What kind of coach do I need?" I decided to invest in a fellow physician. She helped me tremendously and I am forever grateful for the experience.

Today, I am a full-time executive coach working with healthcare leaders. Investing in an executive coach can improve your leadership abilities by helping you to improve your emotional intelligence, authentically connect with those you lead, and understand your leadership strengths all while keeping the patients' interests at the core of what you do.

Continuing medical education is a standard part of every physician's career. Leadership executive coaching is just that.

Aspiring leaders need to develop their understanding of how individuals work together, how teams function, and the dynamics of organizations. You can learn these leadership concepts, and the rest of this book is devoted to showing you how.

The five chapters that follow are about: self-awareness and understanding, emotional intelligence, gratitude, community, and networking and connections.

On the surface, this might seem like a surprising list. Where is the mention of business management?

Yes, good leaders need to understand business. But in healthcare, business considerations need to be seen through the lens of patient care. There are many ways that prospective leaders can learn about business. That knowledge cannot be applied effectively without these "softer" skills.

In order to understand how individuals work together, you must first understand yourself.

Emotional intelligence comes into play both in terms of individual interactions and team interactions. Once you understand yourself, you also need to understand your teammates and colleagues.

Gratitude applies to you and to others. In your own life, gratitude is a source of positivity that can help you deal with adversity. For a leader, gratitude is about acknowledging the contributions of others.

Community is a source of strength when we surround ourselves with people who are on the same page. We will talk about how to nurture this kind of community.

Networking and connections refer to the organizational relationships you will need to develop in order to be an effective leader in the complex world of healthcare.

ADAPTIVE LEADERSHIP

The stressful, evolving world of healthcare demands a particular style of leadership, one that is capable of handling change. The adaptive leadership model introduced by Harvard professors Marty Linsky and Ronald Heifetz fits this bill.

Adaptive leadership is a way to deal with complex challenges when there are no clear answers and no experts to rely on (Heifetz 2009). This is clearly what faces healthcare.

The basic principle of adaptive leadership is that because businesses are constantly changing, leaders need to be able to address existing challenges at the same time that they anticipate, and prepare to deal with, future challenges.

Adaptive leaders also have several other skills that are especially relevant in the healthcare arena:

- They are able to assess risk and decide if a risk is worth taking.

- They welcome feedback and a variety of points of view.

- They are ready for change, able to decide what must be kept and what can be let go, and they can change direction if needed.

- They are able to handle change that requires both technical adjustment and adjustments in organizational culture.

The question is: How do you learn to become an adaptive leader?

The concept of adaptive leadership is so relevant to the field of healthcare that there are master's programs specifically targeted to the field. And there are also ways you can develop these skills on the job.

Some of the key skills you will need to develop are emotional intelligence, the cultivation of a community of like-minded people, diversity, and a learning mindset.

Emotional intelligence (EQ) will help you manage the ups and downs that are inevitable in a dynamic and difficult environment. EQ will help you recover quickly from setbacks. It will also help you read your team well in order to help them adjust and thrive.

A supportive community, especially the community you create in the workplace, provides a safe place to take risks. And when you are in a system like healthcare that requires change, risk is inevitable.

An adaptive leader is someone who can decide what risks are worthwhile to take in terms of trying new things. This leader can also assess if something is working, and if not, is prepared to pivot.

Diversity is a great source of creativity and out-of-the-box thinking. Diversity is especially valuable during times of change when the existing systems are not working and problems need to be solved. Suppose you have a team with a diversity of life experiences and points of view. In that case, you will maximize your ability to look at all sides of an issue and develop innovative solutions.

A learning mindset can be a superpower. The older we get, the more we are afraid to fail. But having something go wrong is not the same as failing. Failing is when you have something go wrong and do not do anything to make it right.

If you are a physician who is interested in learning about leadership, you already have a learning mindset. Take advantage of it!

CHAPTER 4

LEARN TO KNOW YOURSELF

How well do you know yourself?

When I was in college, I learned about the Myers-Briggs Type Indicator (MBTI) test. I wanted to find out if I was an introvert or an extrovert. I so badly wanted to be an extrovert. I wanted to be seen as friendly, outgoing, and well-liked. I remember answering the questions so that I could try to make the test reflect what I wanted.

As I have gotten older, I have gotten more in tune with who I am and what fuels me. Over the past several years, I have had to relearn what it is that allows me to recharge. When I asked myself how I recharge, the answer was that it is when I am by myself. That is when I realized that I am an introvert.

It was only after I learned this about myself that I was easily able to find ways to recharge and refuel my tank.

When I started out as a healthcare leader, I actually thought I knew myself pretty well. I was succeeding as a doctor, and so I felt I was applying my strengths in a productive way. I knew that I could learn. I had good working relationships with my colleagues and staff. But I was running into roadblocks that I did not understand.

ASK YOURSELF ABOUT YOURSELF

I realized that in order to take on a new role as a leader, I needed to learn to know myself as a leader. It was not so much about what I could do as a leader but about having a clear understanding of who I wanted to be and what I could inspire others to do.

I needed to know my strengths and my weaknesses in terms of leadership. I needed to know what was satisfying to me because that was what I would be inclined to pursue.

It is helpful to approach this process in two steps. First, reflect and ask yourself some questions:

- What are my strengths?

- What are my weaknesses?

- How do other people see me—both people I know and people I do not know?

- What kind of person am I at home? At work? With my friends?

- How do I want other people to see me?

- What matters most to me? What are my values?

- What do I enjoy?

TAKE A PERSONALITY ASSESSMENT

After you have done this, look for objective personality and skills assessments. You will want to use something with validated credibility, such as the Myers-Briggs or Interpersonal Skills Test.

The Myers-Briggs is a well-known assessment based on Jungian psychology. The questionnaire defines sixteen personality types using four scales:

- extrovert to introvert
- intuitive to sensing
- feeling to thinking
- perceiving to judging

You can choose to take a certified MBTI assessment (at a relatively low cost), or there are a number of websites that offer free MBTI-like tests. The Truity website offers one at https://www.truity.com/test/type-finder-personality-test-new.

The Interpersonal Skills Test was developed by university researchers in the UK. You can find it at https://www.psychometrictest.org.uk/interpersonal-skills-test/. This test evaluates your skills in five categories in order to describe how you interact with others:

- emotional intelligence
- teamwork
- empathy
- integrity
- social boldness

But remember my Myers-Briggs experience in college? It is easy to try to answer self-tests— consciously or unconsciously—in order to get the results you want. This will skew your feedback, making it less valuable.

It is very instructive to compare your self-assessment with the answers you get from these other sources.

A tool that I find particularly useful in my coaching is the 360-degree assessment. The 360-degree assessment is a performance tool that many businesses use to review annual employee performance. In it, the employee does a self-assessment and also receives feedback from their manager, direct reports, peers, coworkers, and customers.

The 360-degree assessment can be time-consuming. Many employees dislike this type of assessment, especially when feedback is anonymous. If the process is handled poorly, it can be counterproductive. But if handled well, the 360-degree assessment encourages growth, and I have found it to be an invaluable tool to kick off executive coaching.

A case in point is my experience with a client whom I will call Dr. J.

Dr. J contacted me because she was experiencing high turnover within her organization and felt unsatisfied with her ability to deal with the situation as the leader. Dr. J was very goal-oriented and was working hard to achieve these goals. But something was wrong.

After our initial exploratory call, the first thing I recommended for Dr. J was a 360-degree assessment.

Dr. J was initially reluctant. She had experienced this kind of assessment in a previous job, and it had left a bad taste in her mouth. But as we talked, she realized that she needed to get a clearer picture of herself and how she was perceived within her organization; however, she was so scared from her previous assessments that she declined going through with another assessment.

Since we did not have a 360 assessment, it was more challenging to directly address the specific challenges within her role. We did work on developing new habits, such as seeking continuous feedback that would help her improve her areas of weakness, but having the assessment would have expedited this process.

Each time we met, Dr. J, was able to report a series of small wins that reinforced her new behaviors. For example, she noticed that she was getting fewer complaints from her staff. The overall sense of community among the team also increased.

The results? Dr. J's employee retention and satisfaction ratings from colleagues improved. She received a 10 percent salary increase, moving her into a new pay grade.

The 360-degree assessment is not the only technique that can be used, but it certainly can expedite the self-knowledge you gain and your ability to know the specific areas to focus on.

LOOK FOR WORKSHOPS

Good leaders are constantly learning.

You may not have the time to enroll in a business management or healthcare leadership degree program. But it can be very empowering to pursue self-discovery in the company of other like-minded people. Workshops on leadership development offer this kind of opportunity.

Many universities offer short healthcare leadership training workshops or online certification programs. Most are about leadership in general, but there is also an increasing number of classes geared specifically for healthcare leadership.

Workshops and similar group learning experiences will give you the opportunity to learn about and practice various leadership strategies. You will experience first-hand your instinctive approach to leadership, how others react to the choices you make, what works, and how you might do some things differently.

We offer customized leadership workshops at my company, Pocket Bridges. They can be tailored to the organization's needs and desires for change.

BE OBSERVANT

You can learn a lot by observing yourself and those around you.

To start, be aware of what you do and how you react to the things that happen.

Practice active listening so that you are purposeful about and aware of verbal and nonverbal cues. After your interactions with coworkers, reflect on how it went.

Did you communicate your message? How do you know? Did you accurately hear what was said to you? In addition to what was said, did the person's body language indicate that they agreed with you, or were there objections they did not voice?

Make a mental note of what went well. Think about how you might have handled things differently if it did not go well.

Consider your schedule at work. Do you get to appointments on time? Are you able to accomplish what you had planned? How much time do you spend reacting to the events of the day, and how much time are you able to spend on long-range plans? How do these things affect you?

Consider your relationships with your colleagues. Be aware of their reactions and body language when they are talking with you. Ask for feedback from colleagues you respect and trust.

Finally, observe what happens in your typical day. How much time do you spend on work, and how much time is available for your family and personal life? Do you take work home with you? Are you happy with your work-life balance? Everyone needs time to decompress in order to do their best.

MANAGE YOUR STRENGTHS AND WEAKNESSES

The more you know about yourself, the better you will be able to build on your strengths and minimize and manage your weaknesses.

Your strengths are the areas in which you have the greatest potential for growth and success. When you know your strengths, you can use them to achieve your goals as a leader.

But it is important to consider that your weaknesses can be a source of strength, too. This probably seems counterintuitive. But remember, no one is perfect. Your team will recognize your weaknesses even if you do not! So, use that. "How do I use a weakness as a strength?" you may be wondering.

As a leader, you have the power to be able to tap a team member to handle a task that they can do better than you.

This does not mean that you should simply accept your weaknesses and work around them. In the same way that you will want to develop as a leader by playing to your strengths, it is also important to work on improving your skills in areas where you are not strong. This is especially true in terms of interpersonal relationships.

If you have weaknesses in practical or technical areas, you can look for members of your team to help carry the load. But if you have weaknesses in your ability to relate to your team, this will get in the way of your being able to communicate effectively with them.

When you learn to know yourself, you will also learn to recognize behaviors and interactions with others that trigger negative reactions in you. Armed with this knowledge, you can plan in advance for better ways to deal with those people.

Let's take a look at this through the lens of the Myers-Briggs personality types. Imagine that your type is ESTJ (extrovert sensing thinking judging), and one of your team members is an INFP (introvert intuitive feeling perceiving). These types are direct opposites and can often rub each other the wrong way.

If you know this, you can plan how to deal with it. For example, people with the INFP personality type tend to be emotional, and this can be challenging for the more logical and structured ESTJ. So, if you are dealing with a problem that you know will trigger an emotional response, be prepared to listen and empathize. Do not just dictate.

You will probably not be in a situation where you know the Myers-Briggs personality type of every employee and coworker! But if you are knowledgeable about these principles, you can use the information to regulate your own behavior.

I saw the truth of this with a client, Dr. T, who had just taken on the role of the lead physician at a relatively new clinic. Dr. T was new to management, and so he sought out executive coaching services.

The first thing we worked on was self-awareness. It is not fun to focus on your weaknesses, but as you learn more about yourself, you will discover the areas in which you need to grow. Dr. T learned that although he thought he was perceived to be congenial and approachable, his staff saw him as somewhat intimidating.

Since one of Dr. T's important responsibilities was to maintain and improve employee morale, this was a problem. But once Dr. T realized what was going on, we were able to work together to turn the situation around.

CHAPTER 5

THE ROLE OF EMOTIONAL INTELLIGENCE

We have all heard of intelligence quotient, or IQ. The other side of IQ is EQ, the emotional quotient, also known as emotional intelligence.

The concept of emotional intelligence was first proposed in 1990 by researchers John Mayer and Peter Salovey (Landry 2019). This means that it is relatively new in terms of the physician leadership structure in healthcare organizations.

Most doctors who graduated from medical school in 1990 are still practicing today, in 2022. The idea of emotional intelligence was not only *not* part of their education; it had not entered the management lexicon.

Physicians are taught to think logically and rationally in order to make diagnostic and treatment decisions. They must control their emotions in order to deal with the stress of patient care.

It is not surprising that I have heard comments from many older physicians who do not take the "newfangled" concept of emotional intelligence seriously. However, some younger physicians have a similar attitude—not because they have never heard of emotional intelligence, but because it is a skill they have not learned.

This is a problem. According to an article from the Harvard Business School, a study that compared physician leaders who had similar knowledge and technical skill found that the characteristic that distinguished the most high-performing leaders was emotional intelligence (Landry 2019).

I have seen this in my coaching practice. I had one client, Dr. S, who truly thought she understood what emotional intelligence is. But I knew that she needed to do some work in this area because of what she told me about the problems she was having with her colleagues and staff.

One issue was a difficult relationship with the department manager. On a personal level, the two women never seemed to hit it off. Professionally, they seemed to perpetually have misalignments when it came to the clinic's needs as it related to staffing.

For example, in Dr. S's specialty, Dr. S felt it was essential to hire a technician to perform a particular clinical task. The department manager did not see the value of increasing costs by adding a technician and instead wanted to have the role split among several existing members of the team.

We began coaching with this issue. I asked Dr. S to tell me about her interactions with the department manager, both the problem situations and times when things had gone well. I helped her see when she had shown high levels of emotional intelligence as well as low levels of emotional intelligence and how this related to what had happened.

As Dr. S learned about EQ, she was able to consciously think about how she was interacting at work with the department manager and how her actions were being perceived. As a result, Dr. S was better able to appreciate the nuances of how interpersonal relationships relate to emotional intelligence.

She saw that when she made small adjustments, such as taking the time to connect with the department manager rather than simply walking in and making a request, the manager was much more receptive to what Dr. S had to say.

Dr. S did not always get what she wanted! But she was no longer butting heads all the time with her manager. And after this experience, she was willing to further explore how her actions were being perceived in her department.

Unfortunately, emotional intelligence is still largely misunderstood. When the topic of emotional intelligence is brought up to some leaders and physicians, the initial reaction is, "Are you questioning the way I care? Of course I care! I work in healthcare. If I was not emotionally intelligent, I would be in a different field other than healthcare." There is an aversion to discussing the possibility that their EQ could be improved.

Well, this just simply is not the case. Emotional intelligence is not about having emotions and caring. It is about how you assimilate your emotions and relate to others. It is about how you incorporate others' thoughts into the ways you think, act, and respond. These are essential components of leadership.

WHY EMOTIONAL INTELLIGENCE MATTERS

When you think about it, you have seen examples of the fact that IQ is not, by itself, enough for success. IQ is certainly the basis of academic success, but it is not always the person who gets the best grades in school who goes on to lead her division in sales or rises to the leadership of a large corporation.

Success takes both IQ and EQ.

The fact is that humans are not just purely rational beings—they have emotions that guide their decisions at times. Emotional intelligence is a critical attribute for a good leader because it is the source of a leader's social/emotional skills.

Leaders need intelligence and technical capability. It is emotional intelligence, however, that elevates a leader's ability to inspire and manage other people.

This is because our thoughts and emotions are closely meshed. Many thoughts and actions are based on unconscious impulses triggered by emotions.

In order for a leader to deal effectively with others, they must be able to deal with the emotions that are involved. Emotionally intelligent leaders understand their own emotions and the emotions of the people around them. They are able to use that knowledge to control their own behavior, relate to others, influence others, and inspire them.

Emotional intelligence has two faces: internal and external.

Internal emotional intelligence involves self-awareness and self-management. External emotional intelligence involves social awareness and relationship management.

I talked about self-awareness, or self-knowledge, in the preceding chapter. It is the first step in developing leadership skills. Armed with self-awareness, a leader is then able to manage their own emotions.

Self-awareness—knowing yourself—is fundamental because only when you know yourself will you be able to regulate your own emotions and recognize how your emotions influence others.

A leader who is self-aware and capable of self-management is someone who is able to control their own anger and minimize the impact of stress. In their personal life, someone who is emotionally intelligent knows how to take a deep breath instead of exploding with road rage. At work, someone who is emotionally intelligent knows how to stop and think before reacting to a problem.

Perhaps when you were a child and you were upset about something that someone said to you, a loved one said, "Consider the source." What they meant was, think about how that person felt that made them say that to you.

They are helping you to develop emotional intelligence skills.

I do not mean to imply that most people are totally lacking in emotional intelligence. That is not true at all. For example, one thing most of us learned as children is the principle of delayed gratification. The challenge for leaders is that most of us have a lot of room for improvement in the area of emotional intelligence.

Good leaders are not only self-aware and self-regulating; they are also able to apply emotional intelligence to how they deal with others. A person with good EQ can influence others because they are aware of how other people feel. They are aware of the dynamics of different situations. And they are able to use that knowledge to guide their interactions.

At work, a person with emotional intelligence knows how to read a room. They are able to understand and use what they know about other peoples' emotions. A person with EQ understands that when an employee or colleague gets angry, it is usually about them, not you. Often, they think that they should have been able to do better and are angrier about their own mistake than about what actually happened.

It is well worth developing your emotional intelligence because this will lead to more effective communications, improved conflict resolution, and higher employee engagement with your organization's goals.

HOW TO DEVELOP EMOTIONAL INTELLIGENCE

Research by organizational psychologist and executive coach Tasha Eurich reveals that while self-awareness is the basis of successful leadership, only 12–15 percent of people are self-aware (Gordon 2020). Therefore, by inference, less than 85 percent of people are emotionally intelligent.

Luckily, emotional intelligence can be learned.

There are lots of books, videos, and websites about emotional intelligence. Many of the websites include quizzes that you can use by yourself to get a quick reading of your EQ skills. But you will get the best information if you include both your own self-assessment and the opinion of others. After all, the goal of developing emotional intelligence for leaders is to help you work more effectively with others. I have looked into many of these assessments, and my favorite—and in my opinion, the best one—is by Genos.

I am a Genos Emotional Intelligence Practitioner, and I use the Genos assessments to help coach my clients in this arena. The Genos Emotional Intelligence Inventory (EI) was designed for use in the workplace. Unlike the IQ test, which simply gives you a score, the EI delivers actionable recommendations based on your answers to questions about your workplace behaviors, in addition to the answers from those who rated you. There are also leadership development programs available based on the information obtained through the Genos assessments. These programs can be delivered to a team or individually.

Leaders can use this information to improve.

Developing emotional intelligence is, in large part, about gaining control of yourself so that you can influence others in a helpful, positive way. Here are four things you can do to practice.

Reflect Daily

While you are learning leadership skills, it is valuable to spend a little time at the end of every day to do a self-assessment. Think about what happened, how you reacted, how others reacted to you, and the results.

Ask yourself what you did that was effective and why it worked.

Ask yourself what you could have done better in a situation that did not go well. Was there something that happened that prevented you from managing your own emotions? Did you inadvertently do something that triggered a colleague's negative emotions?

When you take the time to think in detail about the interactions that happened in your day, you are preparing yourself to recognize similar situations and handle them well in the future.

Reframe Your Thoughts

Reframing is a technique from cognitive behavioral therapy in which you consciously identify your negative thoughts and "reframe" them in a more positive way.

Some common thought patterns that can lead to negative thinking include: seeing a situation as all-or-nothing, ignoring positive experiences to focus on the negative, jumping to conclusions, and reacting emotionally without thinking a situation through.

When you are experiencing negative emotions at work, it is important for you to recognize the feeling, and instead of sinking into negativity, think concretely about what is going on.

If you are anxious, do not dwell on what could go wrong. Yes, you need to think about that so you can be prepared to deal with it. But also consider what will happen when things go well (you will notice I say "when" instead of "if").

Also, forgive yourself when you do make a mistake. Everyone makes mistakes. That is how we learn. So, when it is over, think about what you can do better the next time in order to reframe what happened as a learning experience.

Identify Your Emotional Triggers

Emotional triggers are things you see or things that happen to which you have a knee-jerk response. Post-traumatic stress disorder (PTSD) is an extreme version of this. Pre-pandemic, PTSD was a documented problem among nurses and other frontline healthcare workers. COVID-19 has made it worse (Baertlein 2021).

Not every emotional trigger rises to the level of PTSD, but these triggers can still interfere with your ability to handle a situation.

I heard a story about a person, let's call her Mary, whose negative emotions were triggered by tattoos. She automatically thought less of anyone she saw who had a visible tattoo. She knew this was what she thought but felt it was okay.

In the winter, Mary's mother slipped on some ice, broke her hip, and had to go into a nursing home. Mary and her mother both particularly liked one of the nurses, Jo. Then one hot summer day, Mary saw the nurse in her short-sleeved street clothes, which revealed a colorful arm sleeve tattoo.

Mary was deeply embarrassed when Jo—seeing Mary's instinctive negative reaction—immediately apologized, explaining that she normally wore long sleeves, but the day was just too hot for that. And Mary realized that she needed to reset her thinking about tattoos.

If you know what triggers knee-jerk emotional responses in yourself, you can use that awareness to gain control.

Positivity

Have you heard the 1940s song by Johnny Mercer and Harold Arlen that includes the refrain:

> You've got to accentuate the positive
> Eliminate the negative

Latch on to the affirmative

Don't mess with Mister In-Between

It is a catchy tune, and the thought is true. If you choose to accentuate the positive, you will be happier, more productive, and better able to handle the inevitable problems that come your way.

I do not mean to be flippant, however. A bad situation deserves the respect of your attention. How else can you address it? But do not be blind to the good. Do not let the negative cripple you.

This is the same as the management principle that recommends that when you are counseling employees to improve their performance, you will get better results if you focus on what they did right than if you focus on what they did wrong.

Focusing on the positive works when you are dealing with staff, and it works when you are dealing with yourself. It will help you prevent your mind from spiraling into counterproductive negativity.

I apply this principle in my coaching. When I am working with clients to improve their leadership skills, we first work to reveal the client's strengths and weaknesses.

It is important to understand both. But when devising strategies and tactics to improve leadership performance, I focus on the client's strengths.

THE IMPORTANCE OF EMOTIONAL INTELLIGENCE WHEN THINGS ARE TOUGH

Emotional intelligence improves your ability to handle difficult situations.

When we experience stress, it is natural to feel anger, fear, or frustration. These emotions send a signal to the brain that triggers what we call "fight-or-flight." This disrupts our thought processes, causing us to react rather than respond.

A fight-or-flight *reaction* is an automatic survival response. It is based on primitive instincts and emotions. A *response*, on the other hand, involves more consideration. It requires reflection and decision-making.

In stressful times, people tend to act more emotionally, and this makes emotional intelligence more important than ever. People with a high degree of emotional intelligence are better able to see and control their own emotions and deal with the emotions of others.

Healthcare has always been a stressful environment, and this has only been exacerbated by COVID-19. Emotional intelligence matters more than ever.

According to studies conducted by the Capgemini Research Institute, 83 percent of organizations said that an emotionally intelligent workforce would be a prerequisite for success in the years to come (Capgemini 2019).

The Capgemini report was focused on the impact of artificial intelligence in the workplace. As routine tasks become more automated, there is even more urgency to ensure that employees and leaders are able to demonstrate the key pillars of emotional intelligence, such as self-awareness, awareness of others, and authenticity. I think this is analogous to the impact of EHRs in healthcare. As technology continues to evolve and advance, it is essential that we have leaders and employees who are able to demonstrate their ability to connect with others so that we can continue to provide the best care for our patients.

Organizations with emotionally intelligent workforces, both employees and leaders, have significantly greater efficiency and productivity, more satisfaction among their employees, and increased market share. Emotionally intelligent employees have better emotional and mental well-being, a reduced fear of job loss, and an increased openness to change. These benefits are highly desired by organizations.

CHAPTER 6

STRENGTH IN GRATITUDE

Gratitude: *noun*
  Essential Meaning of *gratitude*: a
  feeling of appreciation or thanks
  (Merriam-Webster.com Dictionary 2019)

In the previous chapter, I mentioned using positive feedback as a constructive way to counsel your employees to improve their job performance. That is just one aspect of how leaders find strength in gratitude.

Gratitude is important for you both personally and as a leader, and I would like to explore why it matters in both areas.

GRATITUDE IS GOOD FOR YOU

University of California Davis psychologist Robert Emmons' pioneering research into the effects of gratitude has shown that people benefit physically, psychologically, and socially if they practice gratitude for as little as three weeks (Emmons 2010a).

After three weeks, study participants were found to have stronger immune systems, lower blood pressure, and fewer aches and pains. They were more refreshed by sleep. They reported feeling more positive and alert. They felt less lonely and isolated, as well as more outgoing, forgiving, and compassionate.

In short, practicing gratitude made them healthier and better able to cope with the world.

"Practicing" gratitude is what is important. It is not enough to simply feel grateful for something on occasion. The point is to reflect every day on what you are thankful for.

This is because it is easy to get used to the things that are good—to take them for granted. Once that happens, the good things that are no longer new have less intrinsic power to counter the bad things that inevitably happen in the course of a day.

Keep a Gratitude Journal

Emmons particularly recommends cultivating gratitude by keeping a gratitude journal. The journal entry does not need to be long, and you do not need to journal daily, but it is important to be purposeful (J. Marsh 2011).

Here is what Emmons suggests:

- Approach your journaling with the intention of becoming happier.

- Be detailed about one thing instead of listing a lot of things.

- Focus on people.

- Think about gratitude from two perspectives: what you are glad to have and also what you would hate to lose.

- When possible, record things that were surprising or unexpected because these will elicit stronger emotions.

- Do not journal more than once or twice a week.

As a busy physician, I am sure this last instruction is welcome!

It may seem surprising, but journaling just once a week is actually more effective. This is because the act of journaling will not just be routine.

And why write about one thing? When you write about just one thing, you think more deeply about it. You are also more likely to remember what you wrote. When you remember what you wrote about, you will be less inclined to take the things you have journaled about for granted.

Count Your Blessings

My husband and I have two little girls. Before we put them down to sleep, we say a nightly prayer that ends with what we call "God blessings." At the start, it was "God bless Mommy and Daddy and everyone in the whole world." As they got older, we got more specific. Then we added their grandparents, uncles, aunts, cousins, and sometimes people they met during the day.

The blessings actually do two things. They act sort of like counting sheep, calming the girls down for sleep. More importantly, they reminded them that they are part of a large and loving community.

Counting your blessings is like that. The things you list that you are grateful for may not stick in your mind as vividly as what you have journaled about, but the act of remembering them is a daily reminder of what is good in your life. This is important, especially in these stressful times.

I like to count my blessings at night, just before going to sleep. During sleep we dream and our minds process what has happened during the day. Why not make sure the good things are available to the dreaming mind?

Other people prefer to count their blessings in the morning as a way to get themselves off to a good start. Either way works. It is about what is best for you.

Weave Gratitude into Your Life

Robert Emmons' Greater Good website lists eight other actions you can take to practice gratitude (Emmons 2010b):

1. Use the memory of hard times in the past to remind yourself of how much better things are now.

2. Use the Naikan three questions meditation technique. Think about a person in your life and ask yourself:

    a. "What have I received from _____?"

    b. "What have I given to _____?" and

    c. "What troubles and difficulties have I caused _____?"

3. Learn prayers of gratitude from other spiritual traditions.

4. Appreciate the wonders of being human by remembering and being thankful for sensory experiences.

5. Create visual reminders of people or things for which you are thankful. This might be a quote you post on the wall or a photo of someone special to you.

6. Promise to practice gratitude. The act of promising that you will do something, even if just to yourself, makes it more likely that you will follow through.

7. Be mindful of how you use language. Grateful people focus on the contributions of others rather than their own accomplishments.

8. Think creatively about new things that inspire you with gratitude.

It is not necessary to do all of these things every day. You might use them to inspire your journaling, or as prompts in your home or office.

The more ways you have to practice gratitude, the more effective your efforts will be.

Gratitude helps you feel better. It is important to take care of yourself in order to be an effective leader for others.

GRATITUDE MAKES YOU A BETTER LEADER

Emmons defines two aspects of gratitude: "an affirmation of goodness" and "recogniz[ing] the sources of this goodness as being outside of ourselves" (Emmons 2010a).

The ability to recognize and acknowledge the goodness in others is a crucial quality for good leadership.

The 5:1 Rule

You may be familiar with psychologist Dr. John Gottman and his longitudinal study of the difference between happy couples and those who are unhappy.

Dr. Gottman and his associates observed couples who were asked to have a discussion to solve a conflict in their marriage. The interactions were recorded and analyzed. Nine years later, Dr. Gottman was able to predict which couples stayed together with more than 90 percent accuracy (Benson 2017).

He made these predictions based on the discovery that the happy couples had at least five positive interactions for every negative one. He called this the "magic ratio."

I have heard people describe professional relationships as a kind of marriage, and in that light, the 5:1 rule sheds interesting light on the importance of gratitude.

The Power of Appreciation

Researchers from the University of Pennsylvania Wharton School of Business studied two groups of alumni fund-raisers. For the first group, it was business as usual. The director of annual giving kicked off the second group by telling them that she was grateful for their work.

The second group made 50 percent more calls.

Perhaps the reason lies in how appreciation and gratitude affect our brain, triggering strong feelings of reward. And because this area of the brain, the hypothalamus, also affects things like eating and sleeping, the inference can be made that gratitude makes you healthier, contributing to better work performance (Tanner 2020).

Use Simple Courtesy

There is a reason why travelers are told they should at least try to learn how to say "please" and "thank you" in the foreign language when they are traveling to that country. This simple act can make the travel experience much more pleasant because it shows a level of courtesy and respect.

For the same reason, simply saying please and thank you at work can be a powerful tool for a leader.

I have talked with leaders who think they should not have to say please and thank you to people who are "just doing their jobs." Why not? Just because you are supposed to do something does not mean you should be treated with discourtesy or disrespect.

I have talked with leaders who are afraid that saying please and thank you will encourage staff to ask for a raise or some other consideration. Perhaps that is true if you single out just one person for this kind of attention, but being courteous and respectful to everyone should not cause any problems.

When you express your gratitude for a job well done, your staff and colleagues will become more engaged. I am sure we have all had the experience of the little boost you get when someone tells you they like something you have done. Good leaders use this effect to inspire.

Be Authentic with Praise

I should mention here that it is important to be specific in what you say. A simple "thank you" is always appreciated, but an explicit acknowledgment of what was done is much more effective.

Imagine that you had a particularly busy day in the office. The second appointment of the day took more time than expected, and you had to fit in a last-minute appointment for a longtime patient who was very sick.

You could tell your entire team, "Thanks. You did a great job today." Or you might say to the office manager, "You did a good job handling the backlog of patients we saw today," and to the nurse, "Thank you for helping to make sure all of the patients were ready when I got to the exam room."

Specific praise is authentic, and that praise is more meaningful. It lets the person know not only that you are grateful but that you are aware of exactly what they did.

Do Not Wait for the Big Moments

The fact that a day is routine does not mean that nothing happened that is worth complimenting. Whenever you see a member of your team doing something especially good, be sure to let them know.

Make an effort to express your appreciation every day. This might be appreciation for a job well done, appreciation for initiative, or appreciation for how a person's attitude helps everyone else.

And make sure to spread your gratitude around. Compliment your highest achievers, and also compliment the folks who are still learning. As I mentioned earlier, you will get better results by focusing on what someone did right than on what they did wrong.

Provide Opportunities for Growth

In the same way that you aspire to healthcare leadership, your staff will have aspirations for themselves.

If your organization provides educational reimbursement, help people take advantage of those programs. Or perhaps you might assign someone else to attend a conference that you attended last year (most conferences change very little from one year to another, and you may well learn something from hearing the other person's point of view).

Engage with your employees to learn their opinions and ideas. Involve the team so that they will be invested in what you accomplish.

CHAPTER 7

STRENGTH IN COMMUNITY AND MENTORS

One thing you will soon learn as you embrace your role as a healthcare leader is the importance of developing a supportive community of like-minded people.

BUILDING COMMUNITY

There are three ways to develop a community of support: hiring, membership organizations, and building partnerships. In the forthcoming pages, we will dissect each of these.

Hiring

If hiring is one of the responsibilities of your job, hire the best. No leader does it all alone, so you want to look for people who can do that job better than you.

What should healthcare leaders look for when hiring?

If you are looking to fill an entry-level position, you are looking for someone with the requisite training and a strong work ethic. Behavioral-type questions are a good way to assess this, asking open-ended questions about the candidate's experiences and process.

To fill slots that require more experienced people, look for a track record of job growth. Behavioral-type questions are useful here, too, as they give you a chance to learn more about the candidate: what the candidate might do going forward, as well as what they have accomplished in the past.

Be sure to ask each candidate for the position the same questions. This will give you a better basis for evaluation when it is time to make a hiring decision.

Look for candidates who will be a good fit with the other members of your team. In the high-stress environment of healthcare, you want to create a work environment that makes it as easy as possible for people to get along.

Another important consideration is diversity, especially since one of the biggest challenges facing healthcare systems today is the unequal access to healthcare among minorities and the economically disadvantaged.

Leadership Organizations

Get involved in communities of leaders. There may be professional societies or associations in your area that you can join. Now, thanks to the pandemic, many of these organizations have extended their programs online, and so people living and working in remote areas have increased access to the wider professional community.

The American College of Healthcare Executives (ACHE) is a national association with 78 chapters dedicated to supporting healthcare leaders. Its membership includes experienced CEOs, other executives, and physicians. And, in recognition of the need for strong healthcare leadership going forward, it also has a special membership category for healthcare professionals under forty who aspire to leadership.

There are also organizations devoted to other aspects of healthcare leadership, such as:

- **The American Association of Healthcare Administrative Management, which focuses on the business side of healthcare.**

- **The National Association of Health Services Executives, which focuses on the development of Black healthcare leaders.**

- **The American Health Information Management Association focuses on healthcare information technology—a hot topic in a world of EHRs.**

- **The Healthcare Financial Management Association is geared to healthcare leaders in finance and operations.**

- **The National Association of Healthcare Access Management deals with professionals involved in the availability of healthcare and consumer access to it.**

- **The Association for Healthcare Administrative Professionals is focused on issues affecting administrative professionals who support our healthcare systems.**

- **The Health Care Administrators Association focuses on professionals involved in the administration of health insurance.**

- **The American Association of Physician Leadership has a focus on developing physician leaders and physician executives (USAHS 2022).**

All of these organizations provide continuing education opportunities and have conferences and other events throughout the year. You may not want to become a member of each, but at various times during your career, you may benefit from tapping into the expertise of these professional communities.

Partnerships

Rich Litvin is a coach and leadership consultant—a coach of coaches—and I find him to be inspiring. One of the ways he suggests developing a community of support is through building partnerships.

Partnerships are one-to-one relationships in which you and your partner help one another.
Rich Litvin talks about three types of partnership that can nourish you as a leader:

1. "1+1=2 is a partnership. You're a coach, I'm a coach, let's help each other . . .

2. 1+1=3 is a great partnership. You're a great coach, I'm a great coach, let's build a business together . . .

3. 1+1=11 is when you seek out extraordinary partners—but they stay in their Zone of Genius, which allows you to stay in yours" (Litvin 2021).

Where do you find these partnerships? They lie in the way you deal with everyone around you.

As I said earlier, leadership is a team sport, and everyone on your team has the potential to partner with you in developing and delivering the best possible healthcare. Also, when you think of your colleagues as partners rather than simply staff, you will engender increased respect and better job performance.

This was the attitude demonstrated earlier in the story about the video producer who changed the structure of her company's incentive plan. She recognized that everyone in the organization was a partner in creating its success, from the receptionist who answered the phone and greeted clients at the door to the producer/directors who led the teams for each project. That was partnership thinking.

MENTORS AND MENTORING

Mentors are role models who help us grow.

I had several mentors on my road to becoming a physician. There was an anesthesiologist who took care of me when I was a child. He was my first role model in the field of healthcare. Then there were the nurses and physicians whom I observed when I was volunteering at the hospital.

Two of them in particular took the time to answer my many questions.

I do not know anyone who has not benefited from the guidance or advice of someone more experienced who took the time to help.

This is especially true in a field like medicine, where we learn so much outside of the classroom—as interns and then as residents—working alongside more experienced colleagues. You learn the science of medicine in the classroom. You master the art of medicine through the practice of your skills.

Because medical science is advancing so fast and the healthcare system is so in need of change, mentoring is more important than ever. It is a very effective way to share knowledge between specialty silos and among more diverse groups of healthcare professionals.

Mentoring is a two-way street. As you take on the role of a leader, you become a mentor for your staff. In order to grow in your role as a leader, you will also need mentors of your own.

Mentoring Your Staff

Now that you are a leader, one part of your responsibility is mentoring: sharing what you know, listening, and providing a sounding board to help your staff handle the challenges of their jobs.

The immediate thing that comes to mind when you think about mentoring is helping someone to grow in their area of specialty. Perhaps this is a role you took on for an intern during your own residency. When you are dealing with staff members who are doing a job that was yours at one time, you can provide very specific professional guidance and inspiration.

But mentorship relationships can also cross individual job boundaries. For example, when you are dealing with staff members whose jobs you have not done yourself, you have a valuable mentorship role in terms of helping them deal with the organization. You can talk with them, listen to their thought processes, and be a sounding board for them.

This is an ongoing process that requires trust and open communication.

It is essential that mentoring is collaborative rather than directive. This is not a time for you to simply provide the answers. The goal of mentoring is to help the mentee think things through in order to work through challenges on their own.

You may also find that by letting your mentees come up with the answers, you will learn something too.

Finding Mentors of Your Own

One of the most exciting things about growing in your career is the opportunity to work with more and more people who are excellent at what they do. These are your potential mentors.

Reach out. Be creative. You can find mentors in surprising places.

A mentor does not have to be someone who does the same job as you. You may find a mentor in your organization but outside of your specialty who can help you navigate administrative hurdles; or you may find a mentor in another field who has expertise in a skill you admire and would like to learn.

When I was considering the idea of becoming a coach, I talked with a couple of colleagues who had the experience of being coached to find out how coaching helped them. I also contacted a coach I admired who targeted a slightly different coaching clientele to get some expert advice.

Sometimes finding a mentor is as simple as reaching out to share a cup of coffee and talk. Suppose you see someone in your organization whose work you admire or who has had an experience you would like to know more about—ask to talk with them. Come prepared with some specific questions. People like to be appreciated and are generally happy to share what they know.

The simple act of saying things out loud is a great way to learn. It is analogous to writing papers in school.

The process of writing forces you to use the facts you learned in the classroom, processing and synthesizing the information. When you talk with a mentor about a shared topic of interest, something similar happens. You are forced to put into words the ideas that have been floating around unstructured in your head.

These conversations will be the most helpful when you have a specific learning goal in mind and have taken the time to gather your thoughts to prepare. Be sure to follow up, too. Let your mentor know how you benefited from their advice.

Finding a mentor outside of your organization requires a more formal approach.

You might find a mentor through your medical school alumni association. Conferences and workshops held by the various healthcare professional associations can also be great places to find a mentor.

A mentor could be someone whose work you admire in any field that is relevant to you. Or it could be someone whose background is similar to yours and who has dealt successfully with the same challenges that face you.

If your prospective mentor is someone you have met, approach them first in an email.

People who are very accomplished are also very busy. By approaching someone in an email rather than on the phone, you make it easy for them to tell you if they are too busy to meet with you right now.

Be respectful of your prospective mentor's time. Ask for a short meeting, no more than half an hour, either in their office or on the phone.

In your email, remind your prospective mentor briefly who you are. Tell them what you want to learn and be specific about how their experience relates to your goal—for instance, "I am an oncologist at Johnstown Health Clinic, and have been asked to take on leadership responsibilities. I hear wonderful things from patients about Briarwood Health, and I would like to know about what you are doing there and any advice you can give me about making this career move."

If your prospective mentor is someone you do not know, try to find someone you do know who can be a reference to introduce you. If that is not possible, it is okay to send a "cold call" email.

If your initial meeting goes well, only then should you introduce the idea of a more long-term mentorship. The goal is to develop a relationship in which you can get together occasionally to talk about what you are doing, the results of what you have done so far, and what you plan to do next.

A good mentor is a sounding board, a person whose experience is relevant to you and from whom you can get both good advice and honest feedback.

CHAPTER 8

CREATING CONNECTIONS

There is a model of leadership called the meta-leadership framework that was designed for environments such as the complex, dynamic, and changing one of healthcare. It was developed by a social scientist, Leonard Marcus.

Marcus describes meta-leadership like this:

"Meta-leadership has three dimensions. It begins with the person . . . It is who you are as a person. The second dimension is the situation—discerning what is happening and what is to be done. The third dimension is connectivity" (Hersh 2018).

Why is connectivity so important to leadership?

The answer is simply put in an article by Erica Hersh for the Harvard T.H. Chan School of Public Health: in healthcare, "there are so many inter-twined responsibilities, inter-connected decisions, and critical outcomes. No one is really in charge of everything" (Hersh 2018).

In order to be an effective leader in this challenging environment where neither you nor any other single person is in charge, you need to be able to work with other people. To do this, you need to create connections.

The connections you will forge as a healthcare leader branch out in four directions. You will need to connect with:

1. members of your team;

2. your boss;

3. colleagues across your organization; and

4. peers and other stakeholders outside of your organization.

Let's consider the value of creating these connections.

CONNECTING TO MOTIVATE

In the past, there was an assumption about work: employees are hired to do a job, managers (leaders) are hired to supervise and direct. It was assumed to be up to the employee to be motivated to do the job well.

Today we understand that effective leadership is not about knowing what needs to be done and telling people to do it. Leadership is not about your technical skills, although those skills can earn you respect. It is not simply about setting goals and expectations for your team, although you need to do that. Leadership is about your ability to influence and motivate.

A leader's accomplishments are achieved through their teams. Success rests on the leader's ability to influence others. In order to exert this influence, a leader needs to be able to make and leverage meaningful connections with the members of their teams.

Emotional intelligence is at the heart of this.

The first step toward making connections is simply to talk to people. Use your active listening skills. Get to know the other person. Let them get to know you.

Learn where the other person is coming from. Make an effort to find things you have in common.

In healthcare, one thing that everyone has in common is the desire to provide good patient care. With that as a given, what else can you find? This can be anything, such as preferring cats to dogs, having an interest in a new therapeutic technique, liking the same football team, desiring to improve the parking situation for staff working into the night, or having a child in middle school, etc.

Taking the time to get to know the members of your team will allow you to connect with them in terms of what matters to them, not to you. This will help you motivate them to do their best, listen to what you have to say, or buy into something new.

A truly connected leader has the ability to bring out the best in each member of the team and give them the sense that everyone is pulling together to achieve something important.

Making connections also helps when you are dealing with your boss, with colleagues in your organization, and with external stakeholders. These personal connections, combined with the use of emotional intelligence, help you communicate how you are all on the same page.

CONNECTING TO PERSUADE

Connections also help you persuade at times when you have the same goal (providing excellent healthcare) but different strategies and/or tactics in mind.

Persuasion is not the same as motivation. Motivation is about encouragement, giving someone a reason to do something. Persuasion is about convincing someone to go along with you or even change their mind.

In his seminal work, *Influence: The Psychology of Persuasion*, psychologist Robert Cialdini identifies the basic principles that can be applied to persuade someone to agree with you or act as you request.

One of the principles is "liking." People are more inclined to be persuaded by someone they like (Cialdini 2021).

The characteristics that define liking, or likeability, include:

- someone with whom you have something in common
- someone who gives you a meaningful compliment
- someone who shares your goals

Getting to know someone and making connections is how a leader earns likeability.

COMMUNICATION IS KEY

It is very important for leaders to communicate effectively. To do this, they need to communicate in a consistent way.

Consistency in this context does not mean that you cannot change your mind. It refers, instead, to how you speak.

Psychologist Albert Mehrabian, a pioneer in the science of nonverbal communication theory, conducted several experiments that found that when we talk, our messages are communicated in three ways: through the words we use, our tone, and our body language (The British Library 2015).

Based on his experimental results, Mehrabian posited something called the 7-38-55 rule. According to this rule, only 7 percent of a message is conveyed verbally; the remaining meaning is conveyed 38 percent through tone and 55 percent through body language.

Although Mehrabian himself said that his experiments were not sufficient to establish this ratio without question, his work clearly indicates that how you convey your message is at least just as important as what you say.

Mehrabian's experiments were with verbal communication, but I think this work also has relevance to how a leader communicates in writing. You always want to be clear and present your message in an appropriate way.

One particular challenge a leader faces in this regard is when it is necessary to introduce or implement a program that they do not like or that they know their employees will not like. One example is when a company changes its payroll system.

As a physician leader, it may be up to you to manage the change. How you communicate this information to your team will have a huge impact.

You may, for instance, think that you can establish common ground with your staff by letting them know that you, too, do not like the new system. You provide all the necessary information; it is clear from your body language and tone that you think this change is an expensive waste of time.

This strategy will backfire. You will have a hard time getting your team to accept the new system, morale will suffer, and your staff will lose respect for you.

As a leader, it will be up to you to make an effort to understand how your organization will benefit from the new system. You will not need to fill the staff in on all the details, but you will need to present the information to them in a consistent way. And, if you anticipate any particular problems, make an effort in advance to plan how staff can deal with them.

VULNERABILITY

Vulnerability in a leader may seem like an incongruous trait, especially in a field where the "physician hero" has long been the norm.

Being vulnerable as a leader is not about being weak. It is about being human.

In terms of leadership, vulnerability is being able to admit when you are wrong or you do not know the solution.

No one has all the answers all of the time. We all make mistakes—in fact, that is how progress is made.

In these cases, a leader actually exhibits confidence and strength by being vulnerable. If you have enough confidence in yourself to admit when you do not know the answer—if you are willing to be known in that vulnerable way—your team will understand.

They will be able to connect with you in a more authentic way, and you will be better able to connect with them.

People are much more invested in collaboration when they perceive that they have a valuable contribution to make. That cannot happen in an environment where someone else professes to have all the answers.

It is said that the reason the people who love you can hurt you so badly is that they know you so well. Have you ever had your heart crushed in a romantic relationship? In this type of relationship, vulnerabilities are expressed over a period of time. It's the vulnerability that causes the deepness of the sadness. As another example, has a best friend betrayed you? With best friends, vulnerabilities are also expressed over time. Effective leaders extend that kind of vulnerability to the people on their teams. By no means do I mean that you have to express your deepest and darkest fears, but expressing a certain amount of your personal and professional desires or concerns goes a long way in developing a rapport with those with whom you work. This is also a part of developing emotional intelligence.

A leader in healthcare dances a fine balance with the command and control style of leadership. We all know that there are times in medicine when someone needs to step up and lead the team. But that style of leadership is task-specific.

In order to lead and succeed in the world of healthcare, a collaborative, adaptive style of leadership will be required. One of the great benefits of making connections as a leader is the extent to which this interconnectedness fosters productive collaboration.

TRUST

Good leaders are trustworthy. They tell the truth. They follow through on their promises. And they can be counted on to back up their team.

If something goes wrong, a good leader lives by the maxim that "the buck stops here."

Your team will lose confidence in you if they sense that you are willing to throw them under the bus. If something goes wrong, a good leader does not point the finger of blame. A good leader uses the pronoun "we," accepting accountability on the part of the team.

This is not to say that a good leader will not counsel team members if—no, when—mistakes are made. But good leaders do not distance themselves from these situations.

As a leader, you want to give people a solid framework within which to make decisions and take action. Then, trust them to do the job. Follow up with thanks or counsel as needed.

CHAPTER 9

COACHING, NOT DIRECTING

There is a scene in the movie *Hoosiers* that, to me, perfectly illustrates the difference between coaching and directing.

If you have not seen the movie, *Hoosiers* is about a college basketball coach with a checkered past. He comes to a small town in Indiana to teach and also coach the high school basketball team. The town is so small that there are only seven players on the team. Despite all odds, the coach leads the team to win the state championship.

In the climax of the film, with the game on the line, the coach calls a play that would take the ball out of the hands of the star player, using him as a decoy instead. But the team disagrees, and the star player says that he can make the shot. The coach decides to trust his team, the star player scores, and the team wins the championship.

That is the difference between a coaching style of leadership and a directing, or directive, style of leadership.

A leader who is directive is one who articulates a plan, then gives instructions that are to be followed explicitly. This is the type of leader who can become a micromanager.

A leader who coaches also articulates a plan but takes the approach of providing guidance while trusting the members of their team to know and do their jobs.

Both leaders want to achieve success. The difference is that the directive leader puts the burden on themself. They expect to win by crafting the best possible plan and seeing to it that each employee follows the plan. The coaching leader, on the other hand, relies on the team. They craft a plan and then guide the team to execute it, responding appropriately as the situation changes.

By coaching rather than directing, a leader is able to support, inspire, and bring out the best in every member of the team.

It is not enough to simply toss out a problem and say, "Solve it." A leader-coach is part of the team. The role of the leader-coach is to:

- make sure each member of the team has been trained to do their job;

- provide opportunities for growth and development;

- devise strategic plans and tactics to address problems or new situations; and

- engage the team in the development and then the execution of those plans.

This leadership style does not come naturally to everyone, especially in healthcare, where there are many prescriptive procedures.

If you know how to do something in a way that works well for you, it can be very frustrating to watch someone handle the job in a different way. It might be something as simple as having a neat or messy desk. Some people need order; others thrive in chaos. A leader-coach needs to be able to focus on the results.

Leading people is different from following a medical protocol. But I am glad to say there are several strategies you can use to develop the skills to lead in a coaching way.

SET HIGH STANDARDS

One of the most visible things you will do as a leader is model what you expect from your team in terms of quality and quantity. Let them see that you are working hard and holding yourself to high standards.

Be explicit about the organization's goals, your goals, and what quality looks like. There will be goals for each individual and for the team as a whole.

As a physician, you have been in the trenches, and you know how hard everyone is working every day. You cannot expect your team to keep on going if they think that your move into leadership means the pressure is off for you.

When you ask a lot from your team, it is also important that they see that you are working on getting them the resources and support that they need. Show them you are doing all that you can to ensure the success of the team. If you are running into roadblocks, let them know what is happening and strategize together about how to deal with the situation.

And use your experience to show empathy.

People will not always make a big deal about it when a day is rough, but when you see that someone is having a hard time, it can be enough to just ask, "Is everything okay?" Letting the employee know that you understand what they are going through will go a long way.

CREATE A WORK ENVIRONMENT THAT FEELS SAFE

Do your best to eliminate negative office or hospital politics. You want your team to talk, to be engaged with each other. But make it clear that you discourage gossip and blame.

Be fair so that everyone knows they will be held to the same standards of performance and given equivalent opportunities to learn and grow. As the leader, it is your job to assess risk and know when and how to let team members try new things.

When you give corrective feedback, do so in a way that is objective and specific. Be sure to mention the positive, too.

For instance, imagine you are talking to a nurse practitioner on your team. They generally do good work and have great patient relationship skills, but they struggle with getting complete health histories. You might start by saying, "I see that you have a really good rapport with our patients, and I like how you record patients' behavior. But I have noticed some gaps in patients' health histories." Then, instead of saying, "You need to be more thorough," ask them, "What happened?"

One of the most damaging things you can do when giving corrective feedback is to make it personal. Do not interpret; ask.

Usually, when you are counseling an employee through a job performance issue, the employee knows what they did wrong. You do not need to tell them. That just rubs it in. Your goal as a leader coach in these situations is to help the employees articulate what they will do differently the next time.

Also, foster open and honest two-way communication. Make it feel safe for the organization's employees and direct reports to give you feedback, too. Be willing to accept constructive criticism. Ask for the employees' opinions, and if someone has something negative to say, do not take it personally.

Actively listen to what they have to say. Reflect. And then, consider how this feedback can help you do a better job.

People only take the time to give you feedback when they care. They want to stick with a good team.

SHOW GRATITUDE AND BE AVAILABLE

Gratitude is so important that I devoted an entire chapter to the topic. I do not think it is possible to give too much authentic praise. We all like to know that our contributions are being seen and valued.

A leader-coach needs to be there with thanks, offering specific praise when things go well.

It is also important to be there with guidance and advice when there are problems. Make your experience and expertise available. If there is time, try not to simply give the answers. Help people think through the situation and come up with solutions themselves.

You may find that you are surprised and gratified when a teammate's suggestion is a good one. And if this suggestion is different than what you would have done, you have expanded the capabilities of the team.

For example, imagine a physician—call him Dr. R— who runs a midsized medical practice in the Midwest. Dr. R wants to improve performance at the clinic, and so he starts to hold monthly meetings at which he invites each member of the staff to make suggestions to improve the group's overall performance.

At one meeting, his head nurse makes a suggestion. The nurse herself is an excellent communicator. All of the patients like her, and she consistently gets good information during the intake process.

She is aware that the quality of intake information can be inconsistent. And she has been doing some research on her own about how to improve. At this meeting, she presents a simple script that all of the nurses can follow. It is not a word-for-word script (no one wants to be told exactly what to say). Instead, it is a checklist of things to do or say, and it includes several features that are not specifically related to medicine.

For example, the first thing on her list is to greet the patient with a smile. In a hectic doctor's office, with the phone ringing and a waiting room full of patients, it is not always easy to remember to do this. But patients who are waiting in the doctor's office are often anxious, fearful, or sad, and the nurse realizes that a simple smile makes a difference.

The team discusses the nurse's checklist and decides to adopt it. Dr. R is soon starting to get compliments from his patients about their experiences in the office.

If Dr. R had not involved his entire team in improving the clinic's performance, it is likely that he would not have spotted this area for improvement, and this change probably would not have happened.

ENCOURAGE WORK-LIFE BALANCE

Especially in a high-stress environment, it is critical for both you and your team to strike a healthy balance between work and home life.

Part of this is doing your best to work reasonable hours. Part of it involves developing the skills to be able to put aside professional worries when you are at home.

As a leader-coach, you can help your team in both of these areas. This is a lesson I learned early in my career.

One day I was in a meeting with a lead physician, and I was saying that I did not know how I was going to be able to take a vacation because we had so much to do. He said to me, "Rachel, take a vacation. It is essential for your well-being. You need this time to recover so you can come back fresh." We all need vacations and time away to recharge.

HELP EVERYONE SEE THE BIG PICTURE

Each member of your team has daily and short-term goals. It often seems that there is no time to take a breath, so when things are extra busy or stressed, it can be easy to "get lost in the weeds."

An important role you will have as a leader coach is to help the team step back and take a look at the big picture. This is something everyone needs to understand so that the team can all pull together toward the same goals.

One advantage we are assumed to have in healthcare is that everyone understands that the ultimate goal of every organization—whether a large hospital complex, mid-sized clinic, or independent practice—is to provide excellent patient care.

Unfortunately, when you take on a leadership role, you will find—if you have not done so already—that many of the people working on clinical teams do not believe that management (or administration) shares that goal. They see the management/administration, or the business side of medicine, as being in it for the money.

It can especially seem that way when administrative systems consume huge amounts of time, and the pressure is on to increase the patient load.

It has been my experience that almost everyone in healthcare, no matter their role, does want to help provide excellent patient care. The problem is that not everyone shares the same definition of "excellence."

As a physician leader, you can help in two ways.

One way is to communicate the clinical imperatives to businesspeople and administrators. For example, once you understand that management needs to evaluate—measure—performance, you can help craft measurements that are meaningful and helpful to clinicians and management.

You can also communicate necessary business administration goals to clinical teams. To do this, you will need to:

- articulate the mission and values of your organization and goals for the future;

- talk about how you plan to get there and how you will know when you do (those dreaded "measures" of success); and

- make sure everyone understands how they, and the team, can contribute.

SUPPORT EMPLOYEE GROWTH

In my coaching practice, I have heard physicians say that they do not like employee reimbursement programs because they only encourage people to get the company to pay for their school loans and then the physicians move on. That is operating from a place of fear rather than encouragement and respect.

Every organization has turnover. On average, companies experience an 18 percent turnover rate. Most of this turnover is among low performers; the rate for high performers averages 3 percent. Significantly, for nearly 50 percent of people with advanced degrees and those who have children, company culture is especially important for reducing turnover and increasing retention (Holliday 2021).

As a leader, you know how difficult and expensive it is to hire the right people. If you're already in a leadership role, you know how difficult and expensive it is to hire the right people. But statistics show that while 70 percent of employees who are considered at high risk for retention say that they will have to find a new job in order to advance, employees who feel they are growing professionally are 20 percent more likely to be in the same job a year later (Li 2020).

For some employees, job growth will mean moving on—perhaps in order to take on a new role or to move into leadership. There are limited opportunities for this kind of growth in any organization.

But consider that when you accept this kind of growth and are gracious with employees who move on, you will be expanding your network of contacts. For the folks who remain, you can frame their colleague's move to reinforce the idea that your organization is a platform for success.

For employees who do not want to change their job, growth might mean getting a salary increase, opportunities to network with peers, or learning new skills in order to do their current job better.

When you encourage this growth, you will be encouraging the development of both the employee and the organization. Employee satisfaction will be increased, and the employees will be more engaged with the overall success of the organization.

Typically, organization leaders have more access to certain learning opportunities like seminars and conferences. As the leader of the department, you may not enjoy those experiences, but know that participation could be valuable for the organization and staff. So rather than suffer through conferences or simply not attend, consider sharing this task with your learners. Consider giving a chief resident the opportunity to attend a conference of particular interest. Then, have them come back and report their findings during grand rounds. This would be a win-win situation.

THE LEADER-COACH APPROACH WORKS

Many respected healthcare organizations, medical schools, and universities are adopting physician leadership programs and the coaching approach. They include Harvard, Johns Hopkins, Emory, UCLA, Drexel, Carnegie Mellon, Arizona State, and Wharton.

One program in particular that has gotten a lot of attention is at the Cleveland Clinic, one of the nation's most highly regarded medical centers.

The Cleveland Clinic, in fact, has two strong programs to develop leadership skills among their staff physicians—one provides peer-to-peer coaching; the other provides nonphysician coaching. These programs have been shown to increase the well-being of the clinic's physicians and also increase staff retention. As a result of leadership coaching, the Clinic reports saving $84 million in physician turnover costs over the course of a decade (Cheney 2021).

In a research study about the effectiveness of the Cleveland Clinic's leadership development program, physicians who had completed the training were asked to report what they had gained. Ninety percent of the physicians reported that the program improved their leadership performance on a personal level. This included growth in areas like self-awareness, self-management, social awareness, relationship management, and specifically the ability to nurture and develop the abilities of others. The physicians also reported improvements in several organizational areas, including organizational processes, organizational change, patient care, and strategic planning (Mustafa et al. 2019).

Coaching can make a big difference for physicians aspiring to take on their first leadership position and for those who want to advance and improve their skills.

WHAT'S NEXT FOR YOU?

I think it is clear that physicians need to be a part of the conversation as we work to address the challenges that require solutions in the healthcare system. This means that physicians need to be involved in leadership.

The problem is the training you get to become a physician and lead clinical teams is, in many ways, antithetical to the skills you need to be an organizational leader. So as a physician who is stepping into a leadership role, you will probably be in a position to need to learn "on the job."

You can also learn leadership principles from books and online videos. There are academic programs, both in-person and online, that you can pursue to learn management skills. There are specialized master's programs in healthcare management.

The challenge is in being able to practice what you learn and get feedback in a real-world setting, just as you did to hone your medical skills during your internship and residency. That is where coaching comes in.

As you will see on my website, I started working with an executive coach when I began my first leadership position. I learned so much!

My coach helped me reflect on my work as a leader, and I realized how many mistakes I was making in my communications with my team. I learned that I needed to improve my emotional intelligence, leadership, and management skills.

I also saw that many of my colleagues in leadership, lacking experience in medicine, were having trouble understanding and connecting with their physician peers. Some of them reached out to me for help, and I did my best to help them bridge the gap between leaders and physicians.

That was the genesis of my company, Pocket Bridges.

I would like to tell you a story that is so common with executive coaches, especially as it relates to healthcare executive coaches. A physician, Dr. W, was working in a hospital setting and desired assistance with a couple of challenges she was having with her team. She reached out to me for coaching. Here is how our executive coaching sessions might have played out.

Initially, I would perform an introductory interview so that we can get a sense of how Dr. W presents herself as a leader. I would then ask her to tell me what she felt was going well, what she wanted to accomplish professionally and personally, and what she saw as her biggest challenge.

Next, I would complete a couple of assessments: one assessment to clearly articulate what Dr. W's interests are, how she interacts with others, and how she processes and communicates information. The other is a 360-degree assessment that includes key stakeholders. The goal of that assessment would be to evaluate Dr. W's emotional intelligence as a leader.

One common finding that can emerge from these two assessments is the need to address communication issues. For example, let's say that Dr. W has a plan to update some of the policies for one of the surgical units. She may be very enthusiastic about the plan, seeing how it would streamline the workflow for her staff and ultimately reduce administrative costs—but it turns out that she did not communicate effectively to her staff about it.

Specifically, there was a disconnect with addressing the needs of the staff, such as the amount of work necessary to implement the new procedures and policies. Additionally, there was a disconnect with the upper administration about addressing the costs of the project.

It is common for physician leaders to approach a project as though it is a medical diagnosis, not an organizational issue.

The problem here is twofold. First, Dr. W had not included any members of the team in developing the plan.

And then, when she presented the plan, she had not fully considered how either set of stakeholders would react.

In light of this, I would partner with Dr. W to develop a strategy to reintroduce the plan. We would then assess the issues and ways to improve and decide upon a new approach.

An initial course of action would be to plan a meeting that involves the affected physicians and staff. The goal of the meeting would be to make sure they understood all aspects of the new plan, how it would be implemented, and what it would accomplish.

We then could develop a new presentation for upper management that emphasizes the "why" of the desired modification, keeping in mind the mission and values of the organization. In doing this work, Dr. W would involve pertinent physicians, staff, and administration in order to identify and address the needs of all those involved.

This is what I do. I am a physician and an executive coach who helps other physicians, specifically physicians who have moved into leadership positions and want expert help in learning how to best do their jobs and achieve their goals. I also work with those who are interested in moving into leadership roles but aren't quite there yet. Many physicians know that they want to get into leadership, but aren't sure of the best path to get there. I work with these people as well.

Additionally, nonclinical leaders have a special place in my heart. I also do executive coaching for these individuals. In the nonclinical leader training, the experience with working directly with physicians is limited. Coming from that physician background, I offer a unique perspective when working with these individuals.

WHAT IS EXECUTIVE COACHING?

There are many people in the world who call themselves coaches. Some are really consultants who use the word "coach." Others are true coaches, people who guide you to find your own answers to problems and to discern what you ultimately desire in your career or life.

Coaches specialize in different areas. There are career coaches, life coaches, organizational coaches, performance coaches, leadership coaches, and executive coaches.

Coaching is different from mentoring or counseling. Mentoring is a learning relationship between two people, one inexperienced and one expert. Counseling is a therapeutic relationship, largely focused on the past. Coaching is a professional relationship focused on assessing the present and guiding the client to achieve future goals.

Executive coaching will help you improve as a leader. Your coach will help you become aware of your areas for growth, develop new attitudes and skills, and implement these competencies on the job.

THE COACHING PROCESS

Executive coaching is an inquiry-based process that involves guided self-assessment, facilitated learning, setting goals, monitoring progress, and providing feedback. It is a close, confidential relationship in which the coach and client work closely together in order to promote the client's career development.

In order to grow, you must first understand where you are now. You must want to learn. You must be willing to examine all areas of your life. This takes consistent daily effort and reflection. It is a process. It takes time.

The first step is to assess the current situation. Who are you as a leader? How do you see yourself, and how do others see you? What are your skills? What are your weaknesses?

Based on the initial assessment, your coach will work with you to identify your areas for improvement and growth. You will develop a plan, and your coach will be there to monitor your progress.

WHAT CAN POCKET BRIDGES DO FOR YOU?

Pocket Bridges offers coaching plans for individuals and organizations. Ours is a three-part process: assessment, development road map, and implementation.

Assessment

Our assessment process starts with an initial consultation to evaluate your current situation and identify issues that are blocking you from growing as a leader.

This is followed by a 360-degree assessment that provides feedback on your job performance through the eyes of multiple raters: your peers, supervisors, and direct reports. You cannot improve your weaknesses unless you can see them. And it is important to understand what you are doing, not only through self-assessment but also through the eyes of your colleagues and staff.

We will use all of this information to identify specific issues that are preventing you from being the leader you want to be and clarify your goals for growth.

The 360-degree assessment tool on its own can be a valuable exercise for an organization.

There are even assessments that can be applied to entire organizations. For example, the Genos Emotional Intelligence Culture Index can be applied to assess the positive and negative emotions in an organization. It rates ten qualities, including productivity, empowerment, anxiety, and stress. This assessment is quick and provides valuable information on the direction in which an organization wants to go.

Development Road Map

The 360-degree assessment reveals where you are and the challenges you face in your leadership—your areas of weakness. Based on this information, Pocket Bridges will develop a solution to accomplish your goals.

I evaluate each problem and recommend step-by-step methods and techniques that will help you improve in each area.

We will then work together to design an individualized road map for growth. This often involves:

- determining your authentic leadership style;
- improving your emotional intelligence;
- helping you understand the motives and needs of your nonphysician leadership colleagues; and
- improving your communication skills.

Each road map is different, tailored to the specific needs of each client. A typical road map will include a combination of formal and informal training. It spells out the areas for improvement and strengths to be enhanced, incorporating all relevant feedback from the 360-degree assessment.

Formal training may include attendance at workshops, conferences, or seminars, as well as e-learning or other educational programs.

Informal training activities are individualized based on the client's goals and opportunities that present themselves in the workplace.

Implementation

The final step is to work with you as you execute the road map.

It is challenging to change your leadership and communication practices. My goal is to make sure that you have all the support and help you need in order to succeed.

The implementation is an intense period of coaching during which we work on executing the road map and tackling new challenges together.

You will get to test your new leadership skills in structured, on-the-job situations. We will reflect together on your daily interactions and honestly evaluate the results during each coaching session.

Throughout this period, I provide you with live guidance and feedback. My goal is to provide you with expert advice in terms of how to effect change, along with a safe place to practice and learn.

GROWING TOGETHER

It is deeply rewarding for me to work with so many excellent professionals in the field of healthcare, all dedicated to providing top-notch patient care and improving the healthcare system in every way we can. I would be honored to work with you.

CONTACT

If you would like to learn more about Pocket Bridges, please visit my website at www.pocketbridges.com. Use the Contact link to book a free discovery call to find out how coaching can help you.

Or send me an email at info@pocketbridges.com.

REFERENCES

AAMC. "AAMC Report Reinforces Mounting Physician Shortage." AAMC. AAMC, June 11, 2021. https://www.aamc.org/news-insights/press-releases/aamc-report-reinforces-mounting-physician-shortage.

Abelson, Reed. "Doctors Are Calling It Quits Under Stress of the Pandemic." *The New York Times*, November 15, 2020. https://www.nytimes.com/2020/11/15/health/Covid-doctors-nurses-quitting.html.

Arndt, Brian G., John W. Beasley, Michelle D. Watkinson, Jonathan L. Temte, Wen-Jan Tuan, Christine A. Sinsky, and Valerie J. Gilchrist. "Tethered to the EHR: Primary Care Physician Workload Assessment Using EHR Event Log Data and Time-Motion Observations." *The Annals of Family Medicine* 15, no. 5 (2017): 419–26. https://doi.org/10.1370/afm.2121.

Baertlein, Lisa. "Each Covid-19 Surge Poses a Risk for Healthcare Workers: PTSD." Reuters. Thomson Reuters, September 5, 2021. https://www.reuters.com/business/healthcare-pharmaceuticals/each-covid-19-surge-poses-risk-healthcare-workers-ptsd-2021-09-05/.

Behring, S. "What's Causing the American Nursing Shortage?" Healthline. Healthline Media, August 11, 2021. https://www.healthline.com/health/nursing-shortage.

Belk, David. "Medical Malpractice: Myths and Realities." True Cost of Healthcare, March 14, 2020. https://truecostofhealthcare.org/malpractice/.

Benson, Kyle. "The Magic Relationship Ratio, According to Science." The Gottman Institute, October 4, 2017. https://www.gottman.com/blog/the-magic-relationship-ratio-according-science.

CDC. "Health and Economic Costs of Chronic Diseases." Centers for Disease Control and Prevention, January 18, 2022. https://www.cdc.gov/chronicdisease/about/costs/index.htm.

Capgemini, "Emotional Intelligence Report: Demand for emotional intelligence skills soars six fold in response to the rise of AI and automation." Capgemini, October 17, 2019. https://www.capgemini.com/us-en/news/emotional-intelligence-report/.

Cheney, Christopher. "Cleveland Clinic Promotes Coaching Culture for Physicians." HealthLeaders, September 22, 2021. https://www.healthleadersmedia.com/clinical-care/cleveland-clinic-promotes-coaching-culture-physicians.

Cialdini, Robert. "The Science of Persuasion: Seven Principles of Persuasion." Influence at Work, November 9, 2021. https://www.influenceatwork. com/7-principles-of-persuasion/.

Clark, Maria. "The 5 Main Causes of Burnout in Healthcare." Etactics. Etactics, Inc., November 7, 2019. https:// etactics.com/blog/burnout-in-healthcare-causes.

Clore, Gerald L. "Psychology and the Rationality of Emotion." *Modern Theology* 27, no. 2 (2011): 325–38. https:// doi.org/10.1111/j.1468-0025.2010.01679.x.

Donlen, Judy and Janet Puro S. "The Impact of the Medical Malpractice Crisis on OB-GYNs and Patients in Southern New Jersey." *New Jersey Medicine: The Journal of the Medical Society of New Jersey* 100, no. 9 (2003): 12–19. https://pubmed.ncbi.nlm.nih.gov/14556589/.

Dyrbye, Liselotte N., Tait D. Shanafelt, Priscilla R. Gill, Daniel V. Satele, and Colin P. West. "Effect of a Professional Coaching Intervention on the Well-Being and Distress of Physicians." *JAMA Internal Medicine* 179, no. 10 (2019): 1406. https://doi.org/10.1001/ jamainternmed.2019.2425.

Economy, Peter. "This Study of 300,000 Leaders Revealed the Top 10 Traits for Success." Inc, March 30, 2018. https://www.inc.com/peter-economy/this-study-of-300000-businesspeople-revealed-top-10-leader-traits-for-success.html.

Ely, Danielle M. and Anne K. Driscoll. "Infant Mortality in the United States, 2018: Data from the Period Linked Birth/Infant Death File." National Vital Statistics Reports. July 16, 2020, https://cdc.gov/nchs/data/nvsr/nvsr69/nvsr-69-7-508.pdf.

Emmons, Robert. "Why Gratitude is Good." Greater Good. The Greater Good Center at the University of California, Berkley, November 16, 2010a. https://greatergood.berkeley.edu/article/item/why_gratitude_is_good.

Emmons, Robert. "10 Ways to Become More Grateful." Greater Good. The Greater Good Center at the University of California, Berkley, November 17, 2010b. https://greatergood.berkeley.edu/article/item/ten_ways_to_become_more_grateful1/.

Ercolano, Patrick. "Johns Hopkins Experts Propose Business Training Requirement for Med Students." Hub. Johns Hopkins University, March 31, 2017. https://hub.jhu.edu/2017/03/31/med-school-should-require-business-management-classes/.

Flores, Alissa. "Pandemic Burnout: The Toll of COVID-19 on Health Care Workers and Children." Physicians for Human Rights, May 21, 2021. https://phr.org/our-work/resources/pandemic-burnout-the-toll-of-covid-19-on-health-care-workers-and-children.

"From Worst to First: A Physician Success Story." Relias Media, June 1, 2000. https://www.reliasmedia.com/articles/45660-from-worst-to-first-a-physician-success-story.

Ginsberg, Seth D. "5 Ways Insurance Companies Meddle in Your Health Care. *U.S. News & World Report*, July 13, 2017. https://health.usnews.com/health-care/for-better/articles/2017-07-13/5-ways-insurance-companies-meddle-in-your-health-care.

Gordon, Chad. "The Importance of Self-Awareness with Tasha Eurich." The Ken Blanchard Companies, April 29, 2020. https://resources.kenblanchard.com/podcasts/the-importance-of-self-awareness-with-tasha-eurich.

Gunsalus, C. K., Elizabeth A. Luckman, Nicholas C. Burbules, and Robert A. Easter. "The Self-Aware Leader." Inside Higher Ed, August 7, 2019. https://www.insidehighered.com/advice/2019/08/07/importance-understanding-yourself-academic-leader-opinion.

Hajjaj, F. M., M. S. Salek, M. K. A. Basra, and A. Y. Finlay. "Non-Clinical Influences on Clinical Decision-Making: A Major Challenge to Evidence-Based Practice." *Journal of the Royal Society of Medicine* 103, no. 5 (2010): 178–87. https://doi.org/10.1258/jrsm.2010.100104.

Hargett, Charles, Joseph Doty, Jennifer Hauck, Allison Webb, Steven Cook, Nicholas Tsipis, Julie Neumann, Kathryn Andolsek, and Dean Taylor. "Developing a Model for Effective Leadership in Healthcare: A Concept Mapping Approach." *Journal of Healthcare Leadership* Volume 9 (2017): 69–78. https://doi.org/10.2147/jhl.s141664.

Heifetz, Ronald, Alexander Grashow, and Marty Linsky. *The Practice of Adaptive Leadership: Tools and Tactics for Changing Your Organization and the World.* Boston, MA: Harvard Business Press, 2009.

Hersh, Erica. "Leading Through the Complexity of Health Care Change." Harvard T.H. Chan School of Public Health. The President and Fellows of Harvard College, March 15, 2018. https://www.hsph.harvard.edu/ecpe/leading-complexity-health-care-change/.

Holliday, Marc. "50 Employee Turnover Statistics to Know Today." Oracle NetSuite. Oracle, January 5, 2021. https://www.netsuite.com/portal/resource/articles/human-resources/employee-turnover-statistics.shtml.

Hu, Xiaochu, and Michael J. Dill. "Changes in Physician Work Hours and Patterns during the COVID-19 Pandemic." *JAMA Network Open* 4, no. 6 (2021). https://doi.org/10.1001/jamanetworkopen.2021.14386.

Kaplan, Alan S., and Abigail Abongwa. "U.S Hospitals Can No Longer Afford the Burden of Administrative Waste." Healthcare Financial Management Association, August 20, 2020. https://www.hfma.org/topics/financial-sustainability/article/u-s-hospitals-can-no-longer-afford-the-burden-of-administrative-.html.

Landry, Lauren. "Why Emotional Intelligence is Important in Leadership." Business Insights. Harvard Business School Online, April 3, 2019. https://online.hbs.edu/blog/post/emotional-intelligence-in-leadership.

Lee, Thomas H. "Turning Doctors into Leaders." *Harvard Business Review*. Harvard Business Publishing, April 7, 2010. https://hbr.org/2010/04/turning-doctors-into-leaders.

Lee, Woogul, and Johnmarshall Reeve. "Identifying the Neural Substrates of Intrinsic Motivation during Task Performance." *Cognitive, Affective, & Behavioral Neuroscience* 17, no. 5 (2017): 939–53. https://doi.org/10.3758/s13415-017-0524-x.

Litvin, Rich. "3 Awkward Secrets to Success." Rich Litvin, October 20, 2021. https://richlitvin.com/3-awkward-secrets/.

Lyrics Depot. "Accentuate the Positive Lyrics." Accentuate The Positive Lyrics by Johnny Mercer. LyricsDepot.

com. Accessed March 1, 2022. http://www.lyricsdepot. com/johnny-mercer/accentuate-the-positive.html.

McGonagle, Alyssa K., Leslie Schwab, Nancy Yahanda, Heidi Duskey, Nancy Gertz, Lisa Prior, Marianne Roy, and Gila Kriegel. "Coaching for Primary Care Physician Well-Being: A Randomized Trial and Follow-up Analysis." *Journal of Occupational Health Psychology* 25, no. 5 (2020): 297–314. https://doi.org/10.1037/ ocp0000180.

Marsh, Jason. "Tips for Keeping a Gratitude Journal." Greater Good. The Greater Good Center at the University of California, Berkley, November 17, 2011. https://greatergood.berkeley.edu/article/item/ tips_for_keeping_a_gratitude_journal.

"Medscape's 2021 Physician Burnout Report Finds COVID-19 Takes a Toll: Physician Happiness Plunges." BioSpace, January 25, 2021. https://www.biospace. com/article/releases/medscape-s-2021-physician-burnout-report-finds-covid-19-takes-a-toll-physician-happiness-plunges/.

Merriam-Webster.com Dictionary, s.v. "gratitude," accessed March 1, 2022, https://www.merriam-webster. com/dictionary/gratitude.

Mohana, Malini. "The Motivated Mind: Where Our Passion & Creativity Comes From." PsychCentral, May

17, 2016. https://psychcentral.com/lib/the-motivated-mind-where-our-passion-creativity-comes-from#1.

Mustafa, Sultana, Carol F. Farver, S. Beth Bierer, and James K. Stoller. "Impact of a Leadership Development Program for Healthcare Executives: The Cleveland Clinic Experience." *The Journal of Health Administration Education* (Winter 2019). https://www.ingentaconnect.com/contentone/aupha/jhae/2019/00000036/00000001/art00008?crawler=true&mimetype=application/pdf.

NCCIH. "Mind and Body Approaches for Stress and Anxiety: What the Science Says." NCCIH Clinical Digest. NCCIH, April 2020. https://www.nccih.nih.gov/health/providers/digest/mind-and-body-approaches-for-stress-science.

Patel, Deep. "11 Powerful Traits of Successful Leaders." *Forbes*, March 22, 2017. https://www.forbes.com/sites/deeppatel/2017/03/22/11-powerful-traits-of-successful-leaders/?sh=4d3e8188469f.

Patel, Rahul. "Meeting the Unfulfilled Promises of Electronic Health Records." *Forbes*, August 22, 2019. https://www.forbes.com/sites/forbestechcouncil/2019/08/22/meeting-the-unfulfilled-promises-of-electronic-health-records/?sh=8af09df13629.

Saeed, Atetaz, Karlene Cunningham, Richard M. Bloch. (2019 May 15). "Depression and Anxiety Disorders:

Benefits of Exercise, Yoga, and Meditation." *American Family Physician* 99, no. 10 (May 15, 2019): 620–627. www.aafp.org/afp/2019/0515/p620.html.

Sinsky, Christine A., Lee Daugherty Biddison, Aditi Mallick, Anna Legreid Dopp, Jessica Perlo, Lorna Lynn, and Cynthia D. Smith. "Organizational Evidence-Based and Promising Practices for Improving Clinician Well-Being." *NAM Perspectives*, 2020. https://doi.org/10.31478/202011a.

Stoller, James K., Amanda Goodall, and Agnes Baker. "Why the Best Hospitals Are Managed by Doctors." *Harvard Business Review*, December 27, 2016. https://hbr.org/2016/12/why-the-best-hospitals-are-managed-by-doctors.

Tanner, O. C. "The Psychological Effects of Workplace Appreciation and Gratitude." Emergenetics International, December 10, 2020. https://emergenetics.com/blog/workplace-appreciation-gratitude/.

Taylor, Jim. "The Difference Between Reacting and Responding." *Psychology Today*, October 5, 2021. https://www.psychologytoday.com/us/blog/the-power-prime/202110/the-difference-between-reacting-and-responding.

The British Library. "Albert Mehrabian." The British Library, 2015. https://www.bl.uk/people/albert-mehrabian.

Truity. "The TypeFinder Personality Test." Truity, June 9, 2019. https://www.truity.com/test/type-finder-personality-test-new.

USAHS. "8 Professional Associations for Healthcare Administrators." University of St. Augustine for Health Sciences, February 2022. https://www.usa.edu/blog/8-top-national-associations-to-consider-joining-as-a-health-administrator/.

Wofford, Benjamin. "We're Devastatingly Short on Doctors. Why Doesn't the US Just Make More?" *Washingtonian*. Washingtonian Media, April 13, 2020. https://www.washingtonian.com/2020/04/13/were-short-on-healthcare-workers-why-doesnt-the-u-s-just-make-more-doctors/.

ABOUT THE AUTHOR

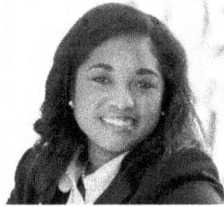

Dr. Rachel Miller is a board-certified obstetrician and gynecologist and the founder of Pocket Bridges, an executive coaching firm. Dr. Miller is passionate about bridging the gap between healthcare leadership and physicians due to her personal and professional life-changing experiences in healthcare.

Dr. Miller earned her bachelor of science in biochemistry at North Carolina State University, her doctor of medicine at the Brody School of Medicine at East Carolina University, and her executive coaching certification from the Center for Executive Coaching. She is also a certified Genos Emotional Intelligence practitioner and a Dr. John Maxwell leadership coach, trainer, and speaker.

Dr. Miller enjoys spending time with her family, traveling, and exercising. She currently resides in Gastonia, North Carolina, with her husband, Casey, and their two daughters, Victoria and Autumn.

To connect, email her at
rachel.miller@pocketbridges.com

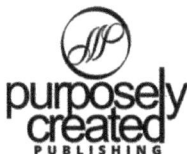

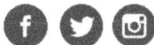

www.ingramcontent.com/pod-product-compliance
Lightning Source LLC
Chambersburg PA
CBHW050731030426
42336CB00012B/1512